My Journey into Alzheimer's Disease

My Journey into ALZHEIMER'S DISEASE

ROBERT DAVIS

with help from his wife, Betty

Tyndale House
Publishers, Inc.,
Wheaton, Illinois

All Scriptures are from *The Holy Bible*, New
International Version, copyright © 1973, 1978, 1984
International Bible Society. Used by permission of
Zondervan Bible Publishers.

Library of Congress Catalog Card Number 88-51599
ISBN 0-8423-4645-7

96 95 94 93 92 91 90
10 9   8   7   6   5   4   3

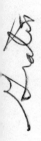

Dedicated to our good friends
Lewis and Amelia Fraser
who have brought so much sunshine
to us all of our lives

CONTENTS

FOREWORD

This is an all-purpose book for people who are hurting.

His doctor told him, "I wish I could tell you that it's cancer. . . ."

By the time that sentence was finished, Bob Davis was introduced to a new world of loneliness, rejection, terror, confusion, misinformation, and termination. It was like walking through the looking glass—suddenly seeing just about everything and everybody from a different viewpoint.

Alzheimer's disease is generally associated with senior citizens. Bob is not old. It is associated with people who have slowed down. Bob had never slowed down. It is primarily associated with loss of memory. But there is so much more about Alzheimer's than the loss of memory.

Because any one of us can have Alzheimer's, it is time to talk about it. This book is not written in technical terms but in gut language so we will understand it.

This book is not really about Alzheimer's but about deep tragedy and victory.

Even if you have no interest whatsoever in Alzheimer's disease, you need to read this book. The insights are so graphic that they provoke us to thoughts we have never had about ourselves.

And this is not a sad book. It is about a man and woman who have been very happily married—and still are. It is about a close family. It is about a vital all-American athlete in a giant's body and with a heart of a child.

This book is about one of the finest men I have ever known on the face of the earth.

BEN HADEN
Chattanooga, Tennessee

INTRODUCTION

Neuropsychology is an outgrowth of expanding knowledge of the relationship between the brain and behavior. By giving a variety of tests, the neuropsychologist can determine from patterns of response on tests where there are deficits in the brain's capacity to function.

Reverend Davis was referred to me for such an evaluation in June of 1987 by his physician. His history revealed a man of considerable intellect and emotional strength, both of which were supported by his strong beliefs in the Lord and his commitment to a life of service in Christ. His recollection of past events was good, but he reported that he was having difficulty with a number of his usual activities, such as reading and remembering, when periods of confusion and disorientation took place.

I began the process of administering the group of tests called the Halsted-Reitan Battery. His scores on those tests that measure remote memory and verbal capacity were quite high, reflecting a higher than average intelligence level. On those tests that show performance on spatial integration, he had some difficulties. He was not able to match blocks to a relatively simple spatial arrangement. When taken together with poor performance on other tests, this is a sign of a general organic deterioration in the brain.

In the middle of one of the subtests, he began to cough. It began first as a slight hack, but the cough increased in intensity over a thirty-second period until he could no longer control his reactions and his body convulsed with each cough. There was nothing I could do but watch.

Within a few minutes he gained his composure. I asked if he was all right. He said yes, and we resumed testing. But he was not all right. He listened to the questions, but he could not answer. For several questions in a row his reply was "I don't know." He was obviously embarrassed by not knowing. I asked him if he understood the questions. He answered that he was not sure and that maybe if I would repeat the questions he could answer them. But he couldn't.

We stopped testing for that day with the plan to pick up the evaluation later in the week.

In those few minutes I saw him deteriorate in a way that I had never seen in any of my previous clinical experience. He went from a cautious but confident patient to a man shocked by the realization that he could not remember or think about some relatively simple questions that he seemed to know that he should be able to answer. My own feeling was one of an empathetic sadness for what he was going through within himself. He knew that what had happened to him was a serious threat to his intellectual integrity. He could not verbalize his feelings, but the look on his face was one of shocked discovery.

When I saw him again he was in the hospital. We finished the testing and I reviewed his medical records, noting that some of the studies had shown some abnormalities in his cerebral blood flow. The test pattern clearly indicated that his brain was not functioning correctly. Though I could not be certain of the cause, there was unmistakable evidence of impaired neurological functioning that was of a general and pervasive nature and that was the result of organic or physical damage to the cells in the brain.

I sent my report to the neurologist and Reverend Davis and I met to review the results. I told him what I had found and what I thought it meant for him. I told him that I did not know the cause, but the pattern of test results would reflect either chronic alcohol use over many years (something we both ruled out quickly), some central nervous system neuropathy due to his diabetes (an unlikely and unusual phenomena), or a form of presenile dementia. The pattern of test results suggested the condition was permanent and irreversible.

We sat for a minute while he digested what I had told him. Then I asked him how he felt about this.

He looked at me with a gentle smile. "I know that the Lord is with me. That knowledge has always given me inner peace. He has always had a purpose for me. I trust that this is a part of that purpose."

This book is about that purpose. It is also about faith and a strong Christian belief. It is about living with a chronic physiological deterioration of the brain's capacity to function. In this book, Reverend Davis has continued to give himself to others by sharing the strength and value of his faith.

Jack T. Tapp, Ph.D., President
Psychological Health Services
South Miami, Florida

PROLOGUE

Alzheimer's disease affects millions of elderly people. Those who are affected by people with the disease are myriad. Some of the latest research estimates report that more than 2.5 million Americans have Alzheimer's disease, and they account for more than 50 percent of all nursing home admissions. Although Alzheimer's disease occurs primarily in older adults, with an estimated 5 percent of those sixty-five years old having it, and 12 percent of those seventy years old affected by it, the disease is not a natural process of aging. It is a distinct organic disease.

Alzheimer's not only devastates the individuals with the disease; it can also ravage families, both psychologically and economically. The psychological upset is enormous, and very little has been written to help families understand and cope. The financial cost of Alzheimer's is devastating, since as of this writing Social Security, Medicare, and many insurance companies refuse to recognize Alzheimer's as a disease that requires skilled nursing care. Without this designation, these programs give no financial assistance for the twenty-four-hour-a-day care necessitated by such symptoms as forgetfulness, incontinence, restlessness, sleeplessness, and wandering, which will devastate a single care giver in a very short time. Perhaps the greatest tragedy is that most of the care givers are elderly mates who barely have the strength to meet their own needs, much less give twenty-four-hour-a-day care to someone else. It is now estimated that caring for Alzheimer's patients costs Americans $40 billion a year, and, with our aging population, that figure is expected to zoom so high as to make it a medical-social problem second only to AIDS.

Sad to say, the family members who love and care suffer the most. Often they are bewildered as to the best way to meet the needs of their afflicted loved one. As Christians who love, they cannot turn their backs on those they love, and as Christians who care, they want to help but do not know how. It becomes especially hard when they are so often, figuratively, slapped in the face by the one they are trying to help and love. Perhaps this book will give some new insights into the confused, fearful mind of the Christian with Alzheimer's.

Alzheimer's affects not only those with the illness, but perhaps affects others even more. Such people include distressed children, mates, pastors, and friends.

For instance, one of the most frequently asked questions among our adults was, "What can I do about my parents? I am here, and they are a thousand miles away. They are becoming unable to care for themselves, and their judgment seems to be impaired. They either ignore me or drive me crazy with their frequent calls. What are they thinking, and how should I react? I just can't understand them. I am at a total loss trying to comprehend their feelings so that I can do my best to help them."

Older husbands and wives often weep at their partner's abrupt and erratic behavior and long for a way to reach inside their loved one's mind to give sunshine and peace. They grieve as suddenly nothing seems to satisfy them.

Pastors wring their hands as, without warning, some of their older members stop coming to church, become furious at them or someone else over some perceived injury, stop their financial support and suddenly transfer to another church, or inexplicably become attracted to a bizarre ministry that last year they would have theologically denounced.

Concerned Christians who work with the elderly become bewildered as suddenly that sweet old saint flares up and hurts them badly. If they have courage to return, they find she is her sweet old self. The next week her fury returns to wound them with a cunning craftiness. Should they ignore her or try to help her?

Friends visit other old friends and discover that on this visit there is another personality living inside that friend's body. They love, and in their love they want to get beneath the surface and perhaps hit the hidden key that will bring their friend back from the moonlight into reality.

Established Christians suddenly weep and cry because they are afraid that God doesn't love them anymore, that they have lost their faith, or that they will somehow miss going to heaven. Must they spend the rest of their lives in this spiritual torture? What can a caring Christian do to break through this blockade of terror and bring assurance back to this troubled mind?

Millions of people have this concern, and there is little written to help them understand or communicate. This is a hidden world because the people so affected have lost their ability to communicate. Even now, as my ability to communicate is rapidly deteriorating, I want to give to the concerned families some insight as to the devastation felt by the Alzheimer patient. Perhaps understanding the "blackness" and "lost" feelings will help families to be more understanding of the unreasonable actions they must deal with.

Betty and I have looked for books and articles to help us understand and prepare and make the best of a very bad situation. We found little help. Even the doctors had little explanation for many of these psychological pains I have suffered. Even if we can't explain the reasons, it helps to know we are not alone. Together with God's help we will accept these "terrors by night," and we will find ways to survive them. The illness may bring changes to our lives and our family—the illness may steal our loved one—the illness may bring sleepless nights and fear-filled days—but my loved one is the victim, not the perpetrator, of this crime.

I want to be the voice for all those victims who lost their ability to communicate even before anyone knew what was bringing on all these devastating changes. Many of these victims were written off by their families as crazy, "fallen from grace," or depressed. I want to shout, "Be gentle with your loved ones. Listen to them. Hear their whispered pain. Touch them. Include them in activity meaningful to them. Help them stay in touch with God. Let them draw from your strength."

I believe then that this book is unique, as I am able to personally express what the countless voiceless people are feeling. As far as I know, nothing like this has been written. Last September as I began to outline thoughts for this book, I was able to write them out. Although many words were missing and many sentences unclear, Betty, my wife for twenty-nine years, was able to decipher my intent and type it into the computer. Then together we read and discussed until I felt sure my feelings were recorded. Chapters 1, 8, 9, and 10 were completed this way. By January I could no longer type a complete thought or keep my head together to write out very much, so I rented a dictaphone and wrenched Chapters 3, 4, and 5 this way. Chapter 7 became so disjointed that we had to take the paragraphs of my description of the physical aspects and let Betty rewrite them. Chapter 6 and the Epilogue are Betty's alone. She has also had a mammoth job to condense my running on and on and repeating myself. Also we have laughed at the many paranoid paragraphs that she has removed as we felt there was no need to so vividly illustrate some of the symptoms I will describe later.

The entire book is a story of a part of my recent personal spiritual journey. That in itself will be helpful to those who have questions about God's provisions, Christ's power to give comfort, the discovery of God's will, the joy that Christ pours on the helpless, the mystery of suffering, and the sustaining peace of the upward look.

ONE
FROM SUNLIGHT
TO MOONLIGHT

Christmas 1986

It was 12:30 A.M. Christmas morning. I was exhausted. I had just finished greeting the last of the 4,123 worshipers who had attended our three Christmas Eve services. My heart was still full of the beauty of the service, the glory of the majesty of Christmas, and the warmth of love that washed over these services.

As I rested against the communion table, I thought again of the miracle of this church. Fourteen years earlier, when I had held my first Christmas Eve service in this new mission work, there were barely a hundred people here. Now after adding over $5 million worth of buildings, reaching our goal of having 2,500 working members, and sharing the load with nineteen other ministers and staff members, we were the largest Protestant church in Miami.

I put my full weight on the edge of the table, closed my eyes and prayed, "O God, the work has been hard but so wonderfully rewarding. Now I pray that we can double in size the next five years and truly be a witness for Christ to dark Miami."

I opened my eyes, looked again at the beautiful sanctuary, and turned around to head for bed to sleep a happy, sunlit sleep.

August 2, 1987

It was 12:30 P.M. I was totally exhausted. My pulpit robe lay on the communion table where I had placed it during the worship service. I leaned against the communion table and wept uncontrollably. The tears cascaded down my already tear-stained face.

Why the tears? Because I had just preached my farewell sermon to the congregation that I loved so dearly. I had just shut the book on this ministry that I felt would soon explode to reach greater heights. The cold fact of the matter was I had just finished preaching the last sermon I would ever preach—at the age of fifty-three.

Why should this happen to me at this time, at the very apex of my career? Had I sinned, lost my faith, betrayed my calling, grown weary of the cross of Christ, or any other such worldly thing? No!

My mind swirled anew as the words of the neurologist echoed on in my head: "I wish I could tell you that you have cancer. There is more chance for recovery. I'm sorry to tell you that you have the Alzheimer's pattern on your PET scan. As you know, Alzheimer's is an irreversible, incurable, terminal disease."

As I thought of Dr. Hochman's words, pain filled me. But then that sweet peace of Christ, which has been so specially given, filled me anew. Leaving the pulpit for the last time, I lifted my shoulders and headed for bed to sleep a shadowy, fearful, moonlight sleep.

What happened from the sunshine and happiness of Christmas Eve to the moonlight and shadowy fears that filled me just seven months later? It was a combination of medical, psychological, mental, and spiritual changes that tossed me around like a cork in the ocean. During this time I had a special mountaintop experience that drew me as close as I have ever been to the sunshine of Christ. During this same time I had the blackest times, in which there was not even any moonlight—times when I was convinced that Christ had forsaken me to be consumed by all the terrors of blackness.

While I still am able to communicate, I want to share this incredible journey into Alzheimer's disease.

Alzheimer's is such a recently named disease that many of the older medical manuals we have around our homes do not list it. It is a disease that causes brain cells to die. As this happens, certain pathways through the brain degenerate, while other pathways are unaffected. The only absolute diagnosis of Alzheimer's disease is by autopsy. However, a nuclear computerized device called PET (positron emission tomography) can show areas of the brain that are no longer being nourished by the blood supply. After extensive testing has ruled out all other possible causes of the symptoms, this test is run. Certain patterns of dead areas are known to be associated with Alzheimer's disease, and a diagnosis is given on the basis of all these very complicated procedures.

I am one of the younger people to be diagnosed as having Alzheimer's. I am also at one of the earliest stages of the disease to be diagnosed. This diagnosis, confirmed by literally hundreds of tests and those black spots on the sophisticated nuclear PET scan, means that now a part of my brain is dead. This condition has an effect on me. For instance, I can no longer remember a list that goes above five items. I sometimes become confused and lost even in familiar stores. I can no longer read even such simple things as long magazine articles. I can become lost in a motel room and not even be able to find the door to the bathroom. All mathematical skills are gone. My mind has become a sieve that can only catch and hold certain random things. My IQ has dropped in half.

Usually, in Alzheimer's disease, the communication skills are among the first to go. I can no longer speak in public, and I shatter psychologically in any pressure situation. Mental and emotional fatigue leave me exhausted and confused. Mental alertness comes now only in waves at random hours of either day or night. However, God in his infinite wisdom has left me with some limited communication skills.

Why has God left me this little window of ability? As I pondered this, I thought that perhaps it happened so that I can be the voice for the voiceless people who suffer from this devastating disease. Perhaps explaining my feelings and emotions will give a glimmer of understanding to those who must care for my fellow-sufferers who can no longer explain their tortured feelings. Perhaps I can still communicate so I can give new hope and assurance to those faithful Christians whose former emotional feelings and blessings are being washed away by the start of this disease, and who are in spiritual despair because they are unable to understand what is happening to them.

Perhaps it is to reaffirm the faith of those who suffer with their loved ones and in their pain doubt as they wonder why God allows tragedy, pain, unfairness, injustice, and suffering.

My wife, Betty, and I have been married for almost thirty years. During this illness our roles have changed. Suddenly she is not only the wife I have loved, but now she is also my care giver. She has to guide me through daily living as I have become a care receiver, unable to fully care for myself.

In the swings of my emotion from sunlight into ever blackening moonlight, her perceptions are constant and comforting to me. Now, let me chronicle the events from the sunshine of that Christmas Day to the moonlight at the close of my pastoral ministry just seven months later—my sudden, unexpected journey into Alzheimer's disease.

TWO
CALLED INTO SUNSHINE
AND SERVANTHOOD

If anyone were to ask me for a one-word description of my relationship to Jesus Christ, I would reply, "Sunshine." The chorus of one of the earliest Sunday school songs I can remember expressed it so well: "Oh there's sunshine, blessed sunshine. . . . There is sunshine in my soul."

To me, internal sunshine, joy, and happiness were synonymous with Jesus. In my rural childhood home setting of farm and church, I thought this experience was something limited to only the less sophisticated and enjoyed only by Christians like ourselves. You can imagine my surprise in my later more enlightened, scholastic years. While studying what I considered to be the cold, logical, somber but theologically correct beliefs of the old staid Presbyterian church, I discovered the opening question in the Larger Catechism of The Westminster Confession of Faith. Question number one asks, "What is the chief and highest end of man?" The answer is, "Man's chief and highest end is to glorify God and fully enjoy Him forever."

"To fully enjoy God!" I felt that I did. In my natural unconverted state I would have been a most unhappy person. The old nature of cynicism, cruelty, selfishness, and the need to win at any price was deep inside me. It was subdued only by the life-changing grace of the Lord Jesus Christ and by the power of the Holy Spirit. I shudder to think what I would be if this old, dark, evil nature were allowed to possess me. It would be the worst kind of darkness.

Jesus Christ not only saved me from hell. He also saved me from this dark, destructive side of my own nature. This na⸱ ⸱ was crucified and replaced by Jesus Christ with a new, optimistic, caring nature, which filled me with sunshine. I lived my life in thanksgiving for the grace of Jesus Christ that set me free from these baser aspects of my old nature and allowed my new nature to soar, to become all that my heart longed to be.

I enjoyed walking in the sunshine of Christ. Much of what determined all of my life's work was the realization that the pure enjoyment of God through Christ was indeed the chief and highest end of man. The motivation for my life's work was to tell all the world of this life-transforming sunshine, wrought by the entrance of Christ into darkened hearts. I yearn for all mankind to discover this sunshine of Christ, which brings the greatest joy to mankind—that is, the full enjoyment of God forever.

The sunshine of Christ did not come to me in all of its brilliance in one single act like the Apostle Paul's Damascus Road experience (Acts 9:1-18). It was not simply the step into salvation, for Christ's salvation was granted to me in a single step as a small child at Sunday school, when I invited him into my heart. Rather, this experience of sunshine was a process of many steps of surrender and renewed spiritual dedication. I have to admit, however, that after each of these spiritual steps I felt at the time that I had discovered all that I could about the riches of Christ's grace and the incredible sunshine that he could bring to the soul.

Entering into the fuller sunshine of Christ was not a cross nor was it some experience of pain or endurance. It was a matter of joy, which developed into an experience of love. As I grew in this love experience with my Savior, I discovered the true meaning of what the Apostle Paul meant when he said, "For Christ's love compels us" (2 Cor. 5:14).

As I continued to enjoy more of the wonders of Christ's love in my own life, I felt a hunger to share this wonderful experience of knowing Christ with others. At the same time, I felt my own inadequacies and my own personal unrealized drives and ambitions.

My father died when I was five years old, and my mother and I, with no place to go, moved back to the home place and the eleven acres remaining from my grandfather's little farm. We had no running water, no central heating, no means of transportation, no work for my mother, and absolutely no money. My mother put out a garden and did day work at any opportunity.

Yet, like many people who grow up in poverty, we had happiness, and most of all we had Jesus, and we had our church. Small matter that we were on the bottom of the sociological scale when we could be one in Christ at church! Even if it meant walking the two miles over the gravel roads in the middle of a blizzard, we were there every time the church doors opened. Except for the times there was serious illness, I can count on both hands the times we missed Sunday morning, Sunday night, prayer meeting, or special services. Church was our life, our joy, our family, and the thing that strengthened us to keep going during the really hard times.

Nevertheless, it is rough growing up in poverty. It produces in a person a tremendous hunger and desire. As I came to the end of my somewhat troubled high school career, I wanted more than anything some of the material things that I had missed all those years.

One truth I discovered was that, despite the words of political documents, God does not create all men equal. He creates men differently. I realized that in spite of our poverty God had given me special advantages that he did not give to everyone. I was gifted with a large, strong body. When I graduated from high school I was 6'7" and weighed 240 pounds. I was also heavily muscled and had the natural ability to excel in certain forms of athletics.

My IQ was well above average, and although I hated being trapped inside a school building, studies came naturally without any effort. I never took a school study book home or did any homework outside of school. Yet, my grades were well above average. I scored at the very top levels of state testing in mathematics. Some teachers said that I was a natural mathematical genius. I could have cared less.

The one attribute that I enjoyed immensely was my ability to quickly read through a book. I read a book a day from seventh grade on. This opened the road to adventure that lay far beyond our worn-out, rocky eastern Ohio farmland.

None of these things was a particular point of pride for me. I had nothing to do with possessing any of these abilities. This was just the way God happened to make me, and I could point with no pride of possession because I had nothing to do with the way I was born. These were just "givens." Only years later did I fully realize that I had a stewardship before God as to how I made use of these "givens."

The only thing I could see when I graduated from high school was that I was incredibly hungry for money. I wanted to put away all the humiliation that lack of money brought with it. I envied those who could go in and buy a soft drink and some potato chips after the team finished playing a football game. For my senior picture I had no suit to wear, and so some of the students, in order not to embarrass the rest of the class, draped and pinned someone's suit coat around my shoulders so that it would look as if I was wearing a suit. We lived in the country and never had a car. As I had the job of cleaning the restrooms after school, and as I also participated in the sports programs after school, I had to walk the several miles home. Poverty either makes a person bitter and angry, or else it gives a tremendous desire to have an abundance of material things. I had that tremendous desire for money. I felt that I would never really be completely fulfilled until I had this desire satiated.

Along with all of these human desires that filled my being, there was also a spiritual desire that filled me. The love of Christ filled me and truly gave me sunshine deep within my soul. It also gave me a burning desire to tell everyone of the happiness of this life. However, in this desire I was completely stymied. I may have been 6' 7" and able to lick almost anyone in a fight, yet I was so terrified to speak publicly that I totally froze. The few times that I tried to speak, I made a complete fool of myself as well as the message that I wanted to communicate. I may have been a mathematical genius, but when it came to the social skills needed to effectively communicate a serious message, I was a real dunce. As I gave myself to hours of introspection, prayer, and serious evaluation, I had to admit that when it came to speaking out for Christ, I was a no-talent person. As far as I could see, my spiritual lot in life was to keep on being faithful to him and to make lots of money so that I could give money to enable the naturally talented people to serve him.

After graduating from high school, I started on my quest for money, cars, and clothes. God in his wisdom gave me all the desires of my heart. I started out driving a truck at a feed mill, and a couple of years and a few jobs later I was a supervisor for Firestone in Akron, Ohio. I was responsible for 121 people and was making more money than I even dreamed of in high school. During this time I had been through eighteen cars as I always traded upward at a profit. I finally acquired the car of my dreams, a beautiful royal blue Chrysler. I have to confess that I loved that car as much as any material thing that I ever had in my life. Much to my surprise, I found that I really did not care that much for clothes, and so that hunger was left behind. Perhaps the most surprising thing was that I found the larger part of the money I was making was given back to the church or Youth for Christ or some mission cause. I could not believe my own actions, especially after having all of this desire bottled up through my teen years.

As so many of these pent-up desires of my teenage poverty were being satisfied, it only intensified my desire to share the love and the sunshine of Christ that filled me. However, even as I had this desire in my heart, my acting upon this desire only brought me more frustration. The longer I worked, the more I became persuaded that I was a no-talent person when it came to doing anything to serve Christ. How I envied those in Youth for Christ who could speak so fluently when giving their testimony about Christ their Savior, or those who could sing or use some musical talent. I even envied those who were saved dramatically out of a life of sin and debauchery and could name the hour of their salvation and how their lives had dramatically changed. I, at least in my own eyes, was a reasonably good person who grew up in the church. There was no doubt of my salvation, but I could not remember the place and hour when it occurred. Neither could I share some "war story" of how bad a sinner I was before I was saved. Quite honestly, I felt a little bad that I did not have a horrible sin record and a dramatic conversion experience like those I heard testifying. I thought if I did then I, too, could have something to say, and thus I could have a definite way to serve Christ. How foolish I was!

I lived like this for two years, and then I heard the sermon that changed my life. The Scripture was a familiar passage from Exodus 7, about God's reassuring Moses that he would be with him while he led the children of Israel out of Egypt. As Moses expressed his fear, God asked him, "What is in your hand?" Moses replied that it was nothing but his rod—just an old stick. God told him to throw the rod down, and it turned into a snake. He then told him to pick the snake up, and then it turned back into a rod. My pastor, known to all as Brother Brumbaugh, further related how God took that ordinary, seemingly useless thing and made it into a mighty instrument for his use. He concluded his sermon by saying that this was how God worked. He could take anything that people would give to him, whatever was in their hand, and transform it to be of great use to him. He then asked us to pray and offer to God whatever was in our hands to be used by him.

As I sat in the pew praying, silently telling God that I was a no-talent person and that there was nothing in my hand, suddenly the Holy Spirit nudged me and said, "What about your car? You have that car, and you can use that car to bring people to church where they can hear the Good News about Jesus. That is what is in your hand!"

I should have been delighted to have an answer to this often-repeated prayer of mine, but I was not. Instead of rejoicing that at last here was something I could do for the service of Christ, I groaned. My car was the absolute fulfillment of my dream. I kept it immaculate. Its royal blue paint gleamed under the many coats of wax that I applied. It was like a beautiful jewel to me, the epitome of my success. Besides that, there was another ulterior motive for not wanting to use my car. By now I was almost over my poverty shyness enough to get up the courage to ask a real girl out—not on a "real date," but perhaps over to Dairy Queen after church.

But this was the call of God to me. "Will you use your car for my service?" With great reluctance I said, "Yes."

But then there came my question, "How?" The answer came back to go out and invite to church this family who lived crowded together in a tumble-down house on a dirt road. I groaned and said, "Lord, they have nine children, with at least two of them sometimes in wet diapers." When you are an only child in bare farm country, nine children seems like half a circus, and wet diapers and muddy roads were unthinkable for my beautiful Chrysler. Yet this was the Lord's direction to me, and, since it came from him, I knew that I must either obey or stop asking for a way to serve him.

The first Sunday morning all nine children came, and I blushed as I pulled into the church parking lot. Yet they were accepted and found friends and a church home. Every Sunday morning and night I went out to pick up this family. Over a period of time, however, most of them lost interest, all but the oldest boy. All this time that I was bringing them to church, I had been praying that God would send around the right speaker or evangelist so that they could meet Jesus and share the same love that I had discovered. Somehow that never seemed to work out. I confess that I argued with God a little bit about that in my nightly prayers. I prayed, "God, I kept my part of the deal and got these children to church, even at the expense of getting up my nerve to invite some beautiful girl to Dairy Queen. Now you have to keep your part of the deal and send in the right evangelist who will touch their hearts so they can get saved."

God never sent the "right" evangelist. He did something better. One night as I was taking the oldest boy, Hollis, home he stopped before he put his hand on the door handle to let himself out. "Bob," he said. "I have been giving it a lot of thought. I have heard all of the preachers talk about being saved, and I have figured out that is the thing I want to do. Bob, I want to get saved tonight—right now. Will you tell me how?"

If he had asked me to fly 200 feet in the air, or turn my Chrysler into a Rolls Royce, I could not have been more surprised. I had been in church all my life, knew the plan of the gospel backwards, and even had memorized all the key verses, but for me to lead someone to Christ, this was over my head. Besides, this was the task of the evangelist, and I wasn't sure a person could actually become saved without going forward or making some kind of a public profession.

I have no idea how long I sat there silently in shock thinking of things like that before Hollis touched my arm and softly said, "Please."

This melted my heart, and, as best I could, I explained how he could ask Jesus into his heart. Hollis hung on to my every word and then asked, "Can I pray this now?" I assured him that he could. In his own words he prayed one of the sweetest prayers I have ever heard as he invited Christ to come into his heart to be his Savior. What a change came over him as the peace of Christ flooded over his being! I will never forget that he reached over and hugged me saying, "Thank you for the greatest thing that ever happened to me."

To say that I was excited would be the understatement of the year. Even though it was past eleven o'clock at night, I can remember going to my friends' homes and getting them out of bed to tell them this exciting news. This was the greatest and most thrilling thing that had ever happened to me. All by myself I had actually led someone to Christ! It was absolutely incredible. If I thought that I had known sunshine in my life and heart before, I now discovered that this was merely the opening rays of a sunrise. At last I had discovered what I really wanted to do with my life. I then began to search for a school that would teach me Bible and how to do this amazing thing better.

When I graduated from high school, I had received various athletic scholarship offers, but I had never considered them because

I hated being locked up in school. I was also totally country, and had no idea how to behave in the upper reaches of society. I kept this in mind as I started my search for a school that would just teach me more Bible, and how to lead people to Christ. After writing for college catalogs from all over the country, I finally chose a college that I had never heard of. The catalog was so humble that I figured a country boy like me would be among friends. It also had a work-study program so that I could earn my way through school. The school was Toccoa Falls Bible College in far off Toccoa Falls, Georgia.

In my newly found freedom from poverty, I had given very little thought to saving for the future. Even though I had earned a lot I had given most of it back to God's work. Now the grim reality that I would be leaving my good-paying job in order to prepare to serve Christ more fully caught me off guard. Financially I was totally unprepared for college.

There was only one asset that I had, and that was my adored big, beautiful, royal blue Chrysler. As the realization spread through me that I would have to give up that one material thing that I adored most in life, I groaned out, "No, God, not that. Anything but that!"

The day came that I had to make my final preparations for school, the day that I had to take my beautiful Chrysler back to the dealer to be sold. This was one of the saddest days in my life, and I wanted to do this alone. Therefore, when I turned the keys over to the dealer, I had to walk back home on the same gravel roads that I had walked so many times during those poverty-ridden days of high school.

I wish I could say that this was an easy two-mile walk home. It was not. As soon as I cleared the houses of the village and reached the open farmland I began to cry. A six-foot seven-inch, 270 pound man walking down a road crying is quite a sight. But I was heartbroken! I said, "God, are you sure that you know what you are doing? Here I am in almost exactly the same condition that I was three years ago in high school!" There was no answer to my desperate prayer.

Grief and loss and pain filled me. I finally stopped walking, turned around and started walking back to the Chrysler dealer. I cried out, "Lord Jesus, this is too much. It is not fair of you to ask me to make this much of a sacrifice. I just am not able to give up my car."

It was at that time I had my first lasting lesson in real servanthood. It was just as if Jesus himself spoke to me and said, "If you cannot give up such a little thing as a car, how can you give up the greater things you will have to give up to be my obedient servant?" That stopped me cold. I thought and prayed for a few minutes, dried my eyes, squared my shoulders, and continued my walk home. After this spiritual decision of surrender a new degree of sunshine that I had never known before filled my soul and life. I was now ready to leave all behind to find my new life at Toccoa Falls Bible College, learning to be an obedient servant to my master, Jesus Christ.

I thought then that this would be the only test of servanthood I would have to endure. Little did I realize that the next major test would occur just two weeks after entering Toccoa Falls Bible College!

I went to Toccoa Falls with very little money. Toccoa Falls had a work-study program in which students could work out most of their school bill. That was good news to me, and I took it at face value. After all, I was a good worker, and I already had proven that I could earn the top dollar. You can imagine the shock when I learned that the pay for their work-study program was seventeen cents an hour, and what was more my work assignment was to be the school plumber's helper.

I thought I had already learned my lesson in servanthood, so I did this new and strange task to the best of my ability. I worked hard in the stifling Georgia heat, putting in the huge pipes for a new steam-heating system. During this time, I began to meet many of my fellow students. Living in a whole world full of dedicated Christians was as close as I had ever come to being in heaven on earth. What was more, there were scores of beautiful, wonderful girls. At last perhaps I could work up the courage to impress some of them, and ask one of them for a real date. This was still an unfulfilled dream in my life.

However, the Lord had an additional step for me to go through in his training school for servanthood. It was an exciting afternoon for all of the students, the afternoon of the big student mixer to be held on the athletic field. All of the students were to be there, and it was a wonderful afternoon of fun, games, and getting acquainted. How I looked forward to this opportunity for getting fully acquainted with the social life of the school, especially with all of those beautiful, soft-spoken southern girls.

But then came that fateful message from my boss, the plumber. The sewer system in the girls' dorm was backed up, and I was to report to him immediately in back of the girls' dorm. That spot was not hard to find. It was adjoining the main road between the campus and the athletic field where the big school social was to be held. As I took off my sports clothes and put on my rough plumber's work outfit, I was heartbroken.

However the worst was yet to come. When I got there the plumber pointed to a big overflowing sewer junction box some twenty feet from the road and said, "This whole system is plugged up. We do not have a pump that will handle it. I'm sorry, but you will have to take a bucket and dip it out by hand so that we can reach the main pipe."

When he said that the whole world seemed to sway, and the trees seemed to become uprooted from the ground. It was the dirtiest, nastiest job that I ever faced. Yet, I always prided myself on being a worker who could handle every task, and so I grimly picked up the bucket and went to work. It was awful! I would dip a while and gag, dip a while and gag. It was only my bullheaded nature that kept me there, and also a somewhat sanctimonious attitude that I was doing this for Jesus.

This was a huge, deep sewer box, and I had been dipping this slime out for about two hours. It was then that the worst thing happened. The social was over. The students started to return, and all those honey-lipped, beautiful southern girls that I wanted so much to meet and impress started to return to their dorm.

The words expressed by the first girl were repeated by every other group of girls that came that way. The first phrase was, "What is that awful smell?" The second phrase was, "What a gruesome mess!" The third unthinking phrase was, "Who is that filthy man down in the sewer?"

The first time that I heard this combination of phrases, anger and humiliation filled me. Never in my life had I been more disappointed and humiliated, and I have to say that, growing up in poverty as the "poor widow's kid," there had been plenty of humiliating times. Big men don't cry, but as I heard these words over and over again, I bent down in my slimy sewer pit and started to sob.

"What are you doing, God?" I cried out. "I gave up everything, even my car, to come here. Now you are ruining my life by taking away my last chance to have any fun. You are just not fair!" With that I threw my bucket down the hill and climbed out of the sewer pit ready to quit. However, as I stood upright in the fresh air my sobbing stopped and my courage returned. I thought that I would finish this job—if nothing else, to prove that I could do it.

Picking up my bucket, I climbed back down into the horrible sewer pit. I started dipping again and retching again. But then came the group of girls that I was particularly interested in. Seeing them before they saw me, I ducked down deep into the sewer pit. Thinking that there was no one around, their remarks were particularly vicious about the "honey-dippers" who would ever do something as filthy as that task.

Needless to say, their remarks totally devastated me. This time when I got out of the sewer pit I threw my slimy bucket as far as I could throw it and said with my face lifted up to heaven, "Lord Jesus, this time it is too much. Three weeks ago I was the boy wonder at Firestone with 121 people under my supervision. I had more money than I could use, the respect of all people, and was driving the car of my dreams. Now I am slimy with sewage, laughed at by everyone, and doing the lowest kind of work. This is the last straw. I am quitting and going back to Ohio where I belong. After all I am just a no-talent person who must have misread your will for my life."

After that prayer there came a remarkable answer from the Lord. Again it was just as if Jesus spoke to me and said, "My child, you said that you would do anything for me. If I cannot trust you to do such a humble thing as dipping out sewers, how can I trust you to do the larger things of life? It is now your choice as to whether or not you will serve me as my obedient servant."

How well I remember dropping to my knees in the middle of that smelly sludge and praying, "Yes, Lord, I will serve you. No matter what the task or how dirty the work, my life is totally dedicated to you to serve you. I want nothing more for my life." After praying that I can remember the sunshine and the joy that filled my soul. This became a bit of hallowed ground for me. I finished my task. My clothes and my body may have been filthy, but my soul was singing as it was filled with more sunshine than I ever knew it was possible to have.

This lesson served me well for the rest of my life. I learned that there is no job that the Lord calls us to that is too dirty or beneath us. When I went to the next college, Taylor University, I also had to work my way through. I bought a garbage truck and earned my way through those two years bearing the ignominious nickname "Tiny Trash." However, this time I did not care. All the sludge from the sewer and all the garbage from the school was nothing compared to the trash and the garbage that I later had to wade through in people's lives as I directed them to the way of the Savior who could by his grace lift them from this mess. What joy and sunshine this later ministry was!

As for the beautiful girls that I so wanted to impress, I never did. This was not all the fault of my circumstances but rather the fact that God had prepared for me a very special girl from Ohio that I would marry five years later, after my graduation from Taylor. Betty completed my life, trained me and balanced me, loved me and gave me the human sunshine that filled me, and shared my great desire to do the Lord's will. In his direction of a life, God has a perfect timetable for all things.

Having taken most of the Bible courses at Toccoa Falls Bible College, I transferred to Taylor University in Upland, Indiana. During my time at Taylor, I majored in psychology, with special training toward working with juvenile delinquents. By this time I had received a definite promise of employment from a large parachurch organization. In fact, they even did a cover story about me in their magazine.

Sports was the major diversion at Taylor. I loved to play football, and by my second season, which was my senior year, I was nationally noted. At the end of the season I was all-conference, all-state, and named to two all-American teams.

As graduation approached, I received two pieces of perplexing news. The first was that the parachurch organization that I had been training to serve suddenly acted as if they had never heard of me, and therefore had no place for me. I was dumbfounded, furious, and totally perplexed at God's direction. The second piece of news was that, in spite of my playing football for a small college, the pros were intensely interested in me. I had inquiries and calls from several major teams, but it was the Baltimore Colts who were particularly interested. I was the same size, inch for inch and pound for pound, as their outstanding lineman, "Big Daddy" Lipscomb.

Feeling that this was my spiritual decision, I told almost no one about this news and the decisions I would have to make. Instead I just returned to my old-time country way of thinking things out and making decisions and went out into the woods for two days just to walk around and pray.

Forgiving and forgetting the parachurch organization that broke its word was easy to do. I have always been forward-looking as I placed my life in God's hands. I realized that he knew more about me than I did myself, and that as my loving heavenly Father he wanted nothing but the best for me as I served him in his chosen place of service. I had no idea what the future held, but I trusted the God who held the future.

The second decision was not nearly so easy to make. What about professional football? Did God close one door so that I would go through this newly opened one? Did not athletes have the greatest opportunity in the world to speak and share their Christian testimony? Was God giving me this generous financial opportunity so that I could pay off my college loans, trade in my threadbare clothes and broken down old car, and get my marriage off to a firm financial start? Everything looked so right!

Yet there was one thing that was wrong. It was a personal thing, yet a thing of conscience to me. I had always regarded Sunday as the Lord's Day, and I refused to work or buy on that day reserved for him. I knew that this was a personal conviction totally disregarded by most Christians, but from my boyhood this was something important to me.

I also thought of how hard it was to get Christians to go to church. Even on the campus of a Christian college like Taylor, I was appalled by the number of students who slept in on Sundays. I thought again that if I were playing football on Sunday, there would be devoted fans who would skip church to come to the game. I would, in effect, be responsible for helping to tear down instead of increasing the church attendance in those areas. I thought of the wonderful Christian professional football players that I admired. I thought and prayed about this for two days. It did not make sense for me to have any reservations, but . . .

After two days of struggling and praying with little explicit leading from the Lord, I finally concluded that this was one of those strange cases of decision-making in the Christian life that I classify as, "Others may; you cannot." In other words, it might be perfectly all right for other fine Christians to do this, but this is not something that I could do and be in the Lord's perfect will.

Humanly speaking, it was with real regret that I prayed and said to my Lord, "I now give up pro football, for I realize that this is not the thing I am to do, but O God, here I am stuck with nothing to do—nothing but to do your will and be your obedient servant."

It was at that moment that the third and highest moment of

Christ's speaking to me and filling my soul with sunshine occurred. It was as if Christ said to me, "You are my special servant. You have chosen me over the world. Trust fully in me and I will lead you in adventurous paths that you never could dream of. Follow me and my distinctive leading, and you will walk in blessing and sunshine."

My path through life was adventurous. After Betty and I were married, God led me to attend United Theological Seminary in Dayton, Ohio. The last thing that either Betty or I ever wanted was to be in the pastorate, but God led us there. I regarded pastors as the "sissies" of Christian service. Somehow I pictured pastors as people who served by sitting in parlors, looking at old photo albums, drinking tea with the ladies of the church, patting little children sweetly on the head, preaching innocuous sermons on Sunday, and finding some silly hobby like growing herbs or golf to fill in all their free time. How wrong I was! God, who in his wisdom knew how I was made and knew my petty, immature thoughts, never limited his call to me as a pastor. The broadened call that I received from God was to be his willing servant. During all the years that I served as a pastor, I could truthfully answer that question, Do you feel that God has called you to pastor this particular church? with an affirmative answer. However, if I were asked if I felt that God called me to the lifelong position of pastor, I would have to answer no. I felt that God called me to the lifelong task of being his obedient servant, whatever that might be and wherever that might take me. By my unique spiritual experiences and by the wonderful way that Christ had led me, I felt that the highest and noblest title was not "pastor" or "minister," but instead "servant of Jesus Christ."

I believe that my entire path from pastoring the Williamsburg Methodist Church in Williamsburg, Indiana, to pastoring the Alto Methodist Church in Kokomo, Indiana, to being the Associate Minister at First Presbyterian Church in Miami, Florida, to pastoring the Hazelwood Presbyterian Church in Hazelwood, North Carolina, and to being the administrative vice-president of Westminster Christian School in Miami, Florida, all led to the place I served for the last fourteen years of my ministry, The Old Cutler Presbyterian Church in Miami, Florida. It was here that I walked in the brightest sunlight that I have ever known, and it was also here that I was submerged into the deepest darkness I have ever experienced.

THREE
THOUGH THE DARKNESS
HIDE ME

I thought that my first few weeks at The Old Cutler Presbyterian Church would be my last. The church was less than six years old, and its few tiny buildings were less than three years old. The founding pastor had just left in a swirl of controversy. When I came in as a substitute pastor to fill the pulpit there were twenty-nine in Sunday school and forty-five in the worship service. When I attended the first meeting of the session, the governing body of elders, the main topic was how to keep from bankruptcy and losing all of the church's property. This was one of the grimmest church situations that I had ever been in, and secretly I was glad I was only the substitute who could walk away from their many problems. I continued to candidate for the larger churches, which I felt my twelve years in ministry had prepared me to serve.

As Sunday followed Sunday at Old Cutler Church, a surprising thing happened. The attendance started to zoom upward. I fell in love with the people, and I believe the feeling was mutual. I began to see great possibilities in this church, and the people began to see that, together with God's guidance, we could make this into a successful, viable church. Some of the people were quite leery of me because I did not fit the mold of the average Presbyterian minister, and I was somewhat leery of the church because this was the smallest church I had ever served, and I had already paid my dues in the years of preparation and experience. However, our great God has the greatest plan, and he led both me and the congregation so that when they extended a call to me to be their pastor, I eagerly accepted.

The Lord blessed the church as it doubled in size and quickly doubled again. There was a continual stream of people coming to know the Lord. It seemed as if the darkness of the sin found in the city of Miami only served to make the light of Christ more beautiful to those who were searching for righteousness and reality. The Lord was truly at work in our midst.

Starting as the only employee, we soon added more staff to meet the needs of our diverse congregation. Our small buildings were inadequate, so we built and built again until eventually we added more than five million dollars' worth of buildings.

The composition of our church was unusual. We were located in one of the wealthier sections of Miami, but from the beginning our congregation took literally the warning in the book of James to give no special consideration to the wealthy or the socially prominent. In any group of members there might be a nationally known company president standing next to a waitress.

Miami is known as a global city, and we were known as the global church. People from all over the world enjoyed the fellowship of our congregation. One Christmas Eve we wanted to reach out to all of the visitors in Miami who might feel alone on this special day, so we gathered all of the people in our church who could speak a language other than English to greet and welcome any visitors who might come. We advertised Merry Christmas in twenty-two languages in the *Miami Herald,* and had our members ready to greet people in any of these twenty-two languages. Yet, in all of our cultural and sociological diversity, we were one in the Lord. There were never any divisions because of our emphasis on Christ above all else.

The church became nationally known as it grew into one of the largest and most unusual Presbyterian churches in America. What was my attitude during this time of growth and fame? I was first and foremost a pastor to my own flock, seldom taking outside speaking engagements and avoiding outside responsibilities whenever possible. My time and energy were consumed in eighteen-hour days right here in my small corner of the world. My attitude was like that of the famous old minister, Charles Spurgeon, who said in effect that he would stay home to sit by his own door and whistle his own tune.

Many people asked me how I handled success. I would lie awake at night laughing at the absurdity of this question. Here I was—a person raised in poverty who had worked for his education by being such noble things as a plumber's helper and a garbage man. I had never in my life even known people who were as successful as some of the ones in my highly educated and successful congregation. These were the last people in the world that I would have thought I could minister to successfully. Only because God put me here was I here. This was not my success. This was the power of God!

Why did our church boom while so many older and more established churches closed their doors in changing Miami? I have no idea. I worked hard. Eighteen-hour days were the norm. My wife and my two daughters loved the Lord, and each worked in the ministry of the church according to their ability or the need. But so did the families of countless other ministers. I studied, not only to present the best biblically-centered sermons and programs that I could, but also to know every sociological trend so that our church could be on the leading edge of community evangelism and outreach. But so did many other ministers. I also led the staff and demanded the best from them for the glory of Christ. I was a strong and visionary administrator and worked to lead by example. Many other ministers did that also. I tried to be there at the hospital or the home when my people needed a pastor. But so did other senior ministers.

As I considered all of these things, I could see that I was not unique. It was not because of any of my particular abilities that the church grew. I could not and did not claim any personal success. This was all from the Lord. I was simply what I have tried to be since my decision at Taylor University not to play professional football—Christ's humble and obedient servant, loving him with my whole heart. Any glory was never mine, but his alone. In fact this was the unofficial theme song of our church, "To God Be the Glory, Great Things He Hath Done."

The feeling I had during this time, which I shared only with those closest to me, was one of joy and sunshine that filled my soul surpassing anything I could ever imagine. I knew that I was in the center of God's will, and there in that special place is contentment, blessing, warmth, communication, and closeness with the Holy Spirit. How I enjoyed my special quiet times when Christ was so real and the Holy Spirit so close that the joy was almost unbearable! It was in these special times of sunshine that I felt I experienced the very essence of heaven itself. This was the secret side of my life that so refreshed and empowered me. These times were too precious to be shared with anyone until now.

The church grew until we had more than twenty-five hundred members and at least that many more who were not members who were served by the church. As always, I was forward looking, and I firmly believed that this was merely the beginning. As I constantly told my congregation, "In today's non-Christian world, Christ is constantly looking for showplaces to demonstrate his life-changing power. By the grace of God, we will be such a place." I was working on a five-year plan that would lay the foundation to add another thousand members in the next five years. We had conquered some of the things that might stunt our growth, and the future looked bright.

It was at this point that my personal world tumbled in. For more than a year I had a persistent, wracking cough and a physical weakness, accompanied by a slight mental loss. Our beloved family physician, Dr. Billy Yeh, was a member of our congregation and took on any illness of mine as a personal challenge. He is an internist and cardiologist with an international practice and reputation. In this illness of mine, he had tried every medicine that he knew could apply. He also had referred me to the best specialists. Still these ailments persisted. It was hoped that this was the result of some obscure viral infection and that my body would eventually fight off the infection and that I would get over it.

There came a day when I was just too weak to move. Mentally, I continued to lose alertness. The most surprising thing was that whenever I exerted myself physically, or whenever I concentrated to study for long periods of time, I would break into long periods of body-wracking coughing. Only medications containing codeine had any positive effect on this debilitating cough. Within a week I was hospitalized.

After a week of testing for all possible reasons for the cough, the pulmonary team declared they could find no physiological reason for the cough from the pulmonary system. They suggested perhaps our cardiologist should look for heart insufficiency. With all leads exhausted through blood, sputum, and pulmonary function studies, it was agreed to do an angiogram in case something had been missed in previous heart studies.

To everyone's surprise, an artery supplying a small portion of my heart was found to be 95 percent blocked. What should be done? After much investigation, my cardiologist made the decision to do an angioplasty to unblock the artery. Normally this area is considered to be insignificant and is left alone, as the risk of this balloon procedure is considered more dangerous than the normal consequence of letting it close. Perhaps because of my size and the unusual position of my heart, this was the culprit. So with great hope and anticipation, the angioplasty was performed.

The greatest shock of my life came after the "balloon" procedure when I reached for a book that I had been looking forward to reading. I picked up the book, and started to read. Suddenly as I was reading on page ten, I realized a stunning fact. I had forgotten what I read earlier and could not even bring to mind what the book was about. I was thunderstruck. As I thought about it, I thought that perhaps this was some of the lingering effects of the anesthesia, and so I put the book down to try the next day.

The next day the same thing happened, and by this time I began to take this condition seriously. I found that I could not even follow the plot of a complicated television movie. I then tried doing the mental mathematics that I sometimes entertained myself with, and I found that too was gone. I began to panic, and so I got a sheet of paper and put down some hypothetical math problems. I discovered that I no longer could even do this. Panic filled me as I realized that unless a miracle happened I would never be the same. In fact, as I thought further about it, I realized that unless a miracle happened my career was gone and my life was ruined. As I lay awake that night in the pain and the shock, I cried and prayed and cried and prayed. Hundreds of others, not even guessing this condition, were praying for me.

The recovery from the surgery and the shock and the pain from discovering this condition so occupied my confused nights and days that I did not realize my greatest loss until several days later. One of the things that I could do with my mind was to be able to remember and almost perfectly visualize any place I had ever been, or any significant situation that I had ever experienced. I did not have a photographic memory by which I could see documents or pages from books as some people can, but I could remember accurately and vividly all the beautiful places that I had seen. This memory was so strong in me that, although Betty and I have traveled widely around the world, I never took photographs. I did not need to. They were in my mind. I would often recall them as I worked on sermons, or at night when I would lie down to go to sleep.

Now, all these pictures were completely gone—erased. I could not even remember what my mother looked like, nor could I picture even the fondest of our family memories that I so cherished. Again, in the privacy of my hospital room, I cried about this loss and prayed fervently that God would at least restore the lovely pictures of my family.

As I continued in further testing and physical recovery, and as the days and nights untangled themselves into a normal hospital routine, I was subjected to the greatest shock of all. Walking with the Lord was not just a pious saying with me. It was a reality that I treasured. The Holy Spirit was not some theological point of argument with me. He was my strengthener, my guide, my comforter, and the one who was with me during my quiet times to point the way to deepen my love relationship with Christ.

For well over thirty-five years, I have enjoyed a very private and very personal relationship with the Trinity. I am not a charismatic who speaks in tongues to enjoy the excitement of the Christian experience. I am a very private Presbyterian who enjoyed the fullness of the Christian experience in my study time and especially in that very wonderful time in the stillness of the night just before I went to sleep. It was then that I worshiped and enjoyed the Lord in our most precious moments. The sunlight of Christ had always filled and thrilled my soul in those drifting moments before sleep carried me away.

Now I discovered the cruelest blow of all. This personal and tender relationship that I had with the Lord was no longer there. This time of love and worship was removed. There were no longer any feelings of peace and joy. I cried out to God for it to be restored. I howled out to the Lord to come back and speak to my spirit as he had done before. This was unfair and unthinkable. I could only cry out bitterly to the Lord, "Why, God, why? How can you leave me at a time like this? Is there some unpardonable sin that I have unconsciously committed? O God, I have lost so much already! How can you take this last joy from me? Why have you made my sunlight turn into moonlight?"

I turned to my Bible to try to get some explanation. It was then I realized fully what my loss of reading ability meant. I tried to bring to my mind the vast portions of Scripture that I had memorized. I then learned how great my memory loss was, as Scripture verses came to mind as if directed by some computer gone berserk, capriciously sending out its own topic at its own timing and not what I was trying to access. I learned that, quite often, the more I thought and tried to recapture the things I knew, the more they scurried away from mental recall.

I left the hospital with a smile on my face to please all those who loved me and prayed for me, but my heart was perhaps in the deepest despair that it had ever known. By sheer stubborn faith, I knew that God was there and that Christ was my Savior. However, the feelings that I had enjoyed all my life were gone.

The hardest time for me was night. I had taken for granted the complexities of the thinking processes. Even going to sleep requires multiple functions of the brain. We make the bodily adjustments so that we will be relaxed and comfortable. After that we turn our mind off so that we can go into that before-sleep feeling of warmth and comfort which precedes sleep.

For as long as I can remember, in this before-sleep state, I used to bring all of the beautiful pictures to my mind. Now they were gone—totally gone.

What was in my mind? Blackness and darkness of the worst kind. As soon as I let go of my concentration to try to fall asleep, there was nothing there. This vacuum was filled with terrifying blackness. Sometimes Betty would hear me crying or even screaming in my sleep. She would hold me, speak soft words of reassurance to gently bring me back to reality. How precious was her touch at those agonizing times!

I was alone, cut off. At those times how I would weep and cry out to God, "Why, God, why? Remember me, I am still your servant. I still love you with all my heart, and I will still serve you with all that I have. Why are you doing this to me? Look at all of the satanic people in the world who are heading millions toward hell, and look at the unfaithful television evangelists who have made Christianity into a laughingstock, and yet you have left them with their minds! Why me? And why this horrible terrifying darkness? What did I ever do to deserve this? Why God?"

As time passed, I ventured out of my home and began to assume some of the easiest duties at church. I could only perform the simplest of my duties, and I could only be there a short time before I had to return home and fall into an exhausted sleep. My staff and my congregation were so loving and patient with me! They, like I, felt that God would fully and totally answer our desperate prayers and that, after adequate rest, I would return to normal.

As I returned to my office for longer and longer periods, I did everything I could to compensate for my devastated mental condition. I carefully tailored reports that I wanted from my staff so that I could understand them and comment on them. I refused to comment on any of the problems that I was undergoing, passing off all questions with a glib answer that every day was getting better and better. I was in the middle of preaching a series of sermons I had prepared several months earlier on a study leave. I postponed appointments and delegated responsibilities that ordinarily I would have joyfully done. In short, I did everything I could to survive, mentally and emotionally, those first weeks out of the hospital.

Deep within me I knew that something was terribly wrong with my mental processes. As I appealed to the teams of doctors they reassured me that time would take care of it, or urged me to accept the fact that I was getting older and I should not expect to be as quick and sharp as I once was. I knew there was something far more seriously wrong with my mind than these surface replies addressed. It was then I requested a neuropsychologist to examine me and my records, and the Lord sent Dr. Jack Tapp into my life.

Dr. Tapp began a search that took him through the hundreds of pages of my medical records and a long interview and testing program with me. I was encouraged by his thoroughness and his attention to my mental changes. His task was a long one that was to last many weeks.

During this time, in order to keep up with my limited ministerial work, I went out of my way to appear happy and cheerful. Emotionally, I was at the point that if anyone had sensed my true internal spiritual struggle and had given me some inspirational spiritual illustrations of how God healed this leader or that, I would have exploded at them with all of the pent-up frustration that filled and occupied my mind. How hypocritical I felt! My overwhelming pain and obsession was the darkness within me—that darkness that made virtually every night into a living hell.

Even if I had every bit of my mental capacity, I still could not have dealt with this inescapable darkness. It was beyond anything that I had ever experienced or imagined. My greatest comfort came by remembering church history and Martin Luther's "dark night of the soul," John Wesley's great depression, and other great leaders of the church who somehow had to endure spiritual blackness of one kind or another. The only reassurance that I had was that for some reason and in some way I was now experiencing this tremendous mind-wrenching experience they mysteriously endured.

In a few weeks, my anger toward God calmed down. My mental condition had not improved but my attitude had. I began to live life moment by moment, and I began to have patience as I waited on God. I still had my secret moments of rage when I lifted my eyes toward heaven and silently screamed, *Why?* but these times happened less and less. Now instead of screaming at God, I found myself beseeching him. That verse from the old hymn "Abide with Me" became the subtle center of my thoughts. The message that I was unconsciously thinking of and the prayer I was always subconsciously praying was, "The darkness deepens; Lord, with me abide." By sheer faith I prayed, "O God, I cannot see you through the darkness that fills my mind and so terrorizes me, but please see me and take care of me in my absolute confusion."

One month after my hospital stay, I was driving the three-mile journey from our house to the church when the unimaginable happened. I was lost! I pulled over to the side of the road, having forgotten my way to the church. As I sat there thinking, coughs wracking my body, I began to have chest pains. At last I remembered that to get to church all I had to do was to keep driving down the road I was on. When I got to church I called Betty, who called the doctor, who immediately put me back into the hospital in intensive care.

The hospital nightmare began again. Soon I was moved out of intensive care and onto the cardiac monitoring floor. Again I was subjected to all sorts of tests looking for pulmonary or cardiological reasons for this cough. Dr. Tapp finished his psychological testing there in the hospital. Now it was decided to look again for a neurological reason for my problems. It was at this time that the Lord sent

Dr. Seth Hochman, who did a most complete and thorough neurological work-up. He and Dr. Tapp worked together under the direction of Dr. Yeh to try to unravel this mystery.

The thing that no one could figure out (or has yet figured out) was the cough. The pulmonary team having previously ruled out allergies, tuberculosis, fungi, bacteria, and viruses decided to try a new inhaler every two days to see if they could fix it even if they couldn't diagnosis it. The strength of some of these inhalers was incredible, and soon I became so weak that I could hardly walk to the bathroom. My mind was constantly fuzzy. As soon as it would start to clear, a new round of medication would numb it. During this time I also was wheeled down to be tested by virtually every test possible. I was CAT-scanned, X-rayed, M.R.I. scanned, and every type of body fluid was tested and retested. Still nothing definitive was found.

At the end of ten days I was released from the hospital so weak I could barely get into the car. Yet home was such a pleasant place to be—until the phone started ringing. Thousands of people from around the country were praying for us. No one could have had greater prayer support than I did, and although I was unable to express myself adequately, no one could have appreciated it more. The exasperating trouble with all of these phone calls was that all the concerned people asked one great question, "What is the diagnosis?" The trouble was that there was no diagnosis. The more that Betty explained this, the more disturbed and angry I became.

Why should there not be a diagnosis? After all, this is the age of miracle medicine. After spending weeks in the hospital and almost $40,000, the very least they could do was to come up with a positive diagnosis! All this time and money and I was still lost in confusion and darkness.

Finally I could stand it no longer. I shouted at Betty, "I have had enough. If they do not have a diagnosis, why am I using these inhalers and medicine that are about killing me? If I am going to die, I would just as soon die natural and comfortable. Let's leave all of the unessential medicine behind, and let's leave all the doctors and hospitals behind, and let's leave the telephone and all the unanswerable questions behind, and let's just get in the car, and even if we only drive fifty miles a day let's just leave and head for the West."

Betty just lovingly looked at me twice and said, "OK, honey," and began to pack the suitcases for our trip west. What a woman!

FOUR
THE REACHING POWER
OF CHRIST

As we headed west, my body gradually began to gain strength. I was able to stay awake several hours a day. Gradually my physical strength returned so that I was able to leave the car and walk to the various roadside points of interest.

My spiritual life was still most miserable. I could not read the Bible. I could not pray as I wanted because my emotions were dead and cut off. There was no feedback from God the Holy Spirit. As I tried to fall asleep only blackness and misery came, misery so terrifying that I could not drop off to sleep. Nighttime was horrible. My mind could not rest and grow calm but instead raced relentlessly, thinking dreadful thoughts of despair. Invariably I lay there, terrified by a darkness that I could not understand.

My mind also raced about, grasping for the comfort of the Savior whom I knew and loved and for the emotional peace that he could give me, but finding nothing. I concluded that the only reason for such darkness must be spiritual. Unnamed guilt filled me. Yet the only guilt I could put a name to was failure to read my Bible. But I could not read, and would God condemn me for this? I could only lie there and cry, "Oh God, why? Why?"

"If I cannot find fellowship and joy again, what will happen to my professional life? I cannot lead Christ's church into light and truth when I am full of darkness." Why would God allow this to happen at the height of my effectiveness in the ministry? I had given my entire life to become the best pastor I could possibly be. The thought of total retirement had never crossed my mind. I felt that if I should leave the pastorate I would teach in seminary and pass on the things that I had learned to those younger men preparing for the ministry. I had also considered leading in church training organizations to show how to make churches grow in unusual situations. For years one of my favorite expressions had been, "God has no retirement plan." Retirement from Christian service had never entered my mind. But now everything that I had given myself for and studied for these past years was gone, lost in the dark recesses of my mind. As I thought of the sheer waste of this, I groaned out "Why, God? Why?"

In addition to all of these things, there was the plain fear of the unknown. At this time I had no idea whether this was a psychological breakdown, a result of some organic disease that could be cured, or some rare unknown thing that would just lead me downward into complete physical and mental devastation. I had no idea what the consequences of my illness would be, and if it would totally destroy me and my family.

Feasting my eyes on the ever-changing scenery caused me to praise God for the wonder of his creation. The trip became more and more enjoyable as my physical strength returned to normal. During the day, I could praise God as I had reminders to lead my thoughts heavenward. But at night when I could no longer look upon God's handiwork, the darkness returned perhaps magnified by contrast to the grandeur of the day. At night I cried out to Christ by the hour. Why had he deserted me in this, my greatest time of need?

One night in Wyoming, as I lay in a motel crying out to my Lord, my long desperate prayers were suddenly answered. As I lay there in the blackness silently shrieking out my often repeated prayer, there was suddenly a light that seemed to fill my very soul. The sweet, holy presence of Christ came to me. He spoke to my spirit and said,

"Take my peace. Stop your struggling. It is all right. This is all in keeping with my will for your life. I now release you from the burden of the heavy yoke of pastoring that I placed upon you. Relax and stop struggling in your desperate search for answers. I will hold you. Lie back in your Shepherd's arms, and take my peace."

What a precious moment this was! At last all my prayers that I had cried out to Christ over the past few weeks were answered in the most complete and precious way that I knew possible. My spiritual and emotional needs had been fully and completely met. I lay in bed and cried like a baby. At last I had my inner pain and rage pacified, and I had all those perplexing inner spiritual questions answered. Furthermore, I had a new direction in life and a peace and release that allowed me to face the world with the absolute answer of, "Yes, it is all true. All that I have preached about the supernatural peace of Christ is true. At last this tremendous peace of Christ has transformed the deepest part of me. Now I can again speak about the peace and the power of Christ without the slightest trace of hypocrisy."

In my confused and shattered emotional and mental condition, Christ had to meet me in this special way. He adjusted his way of comforting me so that it would immerse me in the radiance of his very presence. I do not believe there was ever before a time in my life when I needed this kind of miracle. Ever since my salvation experience, I could always reach up to Jesus. Now in my helplessness he reached down to me. His love overwhelmed me as he told me to take and enjoy his peace, and that the yoke of the pastoral ministry that had obsessed me and driven me on to deeper and greater service was now lifted from my shoulders. My new and simple service to him was to rest in him and moment by moment take his peace and use his strength to simply live.

When I awoke the next morning, the winds of confusion and frustration about all the "whys" in my life were gone. The very presence and peace of Christ absolutely overflowed me deep inside, and I had been changed. I discovered in a richer way than I ever knew possible the peace that surpasses all understanding Jesus promised. Now, instead of my reaching out to Christ by prayer, intellectual determination, sheer bull-headed faith, or by aggressively claiming the promises of Scripture, Christ reached down and held me close to him. The only way I can describe it is that my Good Shepherd took me, his special lamb, in his arms and cuddled me close. As he cuddled me he assured me that this was all in his will. I could now rest from my struggles, enjoy my daily life as it came, and have his peace. From now on, my lot in life would be to be especially held by the Shepherd, letting him fully care for me.

The frustration, pain, aggravation, or irrational thinking did not leave immediately. The old saying that, "God did not promise us smooth seas but a safe harbor," is especially meaningful to me now. Life is never a simple all good or all bad experience. Pain and pleasure, sorrow and joy, mingle in the rope of life for all people, the whole and handicapped alike.

This experience that finally lifted the dark veil for a brief moment did not make my brain whole again. I am still handicapped and will continue to become more and more dependent as my disease progresses. But in my darkness I am again assured that I am not alone. As Isaiah 43:2 reminds us of God's words, "When you pass through the waters, I will be with you; and when you pass through the rivers, they will not sweep over you."

I still have the aggravations of daily living. For instance, it is annoying to be unable to remember information such as my license tag. It is embarrassing and irritating to go to a service station and have to make two trips back to the car to check the license plate because I forgot the number between the pump and the cash register. How frightening it is to go into a large, familiar shopping center with crowds and blinking lights and become totally lost! How humiliating it is to be unable to make the right change and ask the cashier to pick the correct coins from my hand!

It is still sometimes terrifying at night. When I let my mind go in order to go to sleep, my mind still slips into blankness and moonlight. However, this is all just surface frustration, brought on by the constant process of losing control at the daily living level. I can either struggle angrily and uselessly against the inevitable, or else I can admit my inadequacy and humbly ask for help. I choose to do the latter and keep a calmer and more peaceful mind. Fortunately, I can still make this choice, but it is possible with the progress of the brain damage that I will lose this ability.

I must learn a new life-style, accommodating to my limitations to reduce the irritation and frustration of constant failure. I must stay in my limited familiar surroundings or go in absolute blind trust with someone who will take care of me. Many of my old activities are gone forever. Emotionally this is difficult. I naturally mourn the loss of old abilities and skills that are now suddenly gone. I try to focus my attention on the things I can still do and enjoy. For instance, the recorded books for the blind supplied by the Library of Congress have filled the tremendous void left by the inability to read. In my personal emotional struggle, I find that a visit to a rest home increases my gratitude immensely and helps me bring the parameters of my present life into proper perspective. The old Indian proverb expresses this well, "I complained because I had no moccasins until I met a man who had no feet."

I am learning to take strength and comfort wherever and whenever it comes to me. Since it is no longer possible to feed my inner man through the usual channels of prayer, meditation, and Bible study, I am learning to be strengthened by words and instructions that suddenly pop into my mind. To recall definite things, particularly under stress, is very difficult. Somehow the more I try to think of something, the more the thoughts disappear. However, at times certain things pop into my mind, much to my surprise and everyone else's. I cannot read the Bible, but suddenly miscellaneous Bible verses come to mind. I take these and think about them for as long as I can, enjoying their truths and praising God for this facet of blessing. As I do this, I also have a reason to thank God for his goodness.

I have a life that can be either frustrating and frightening or peaceful and submissive. The choice is mine. I choose to take things moment by moment, thankful for everything that I have, instead of raging wildly at the things that I have lost. I must thank God for the ability to do this. I know there must be many people who would like to do this, but in their illness they have lost the power to concentrate enough to make this choice.

In accepting this progressive handicap as from the Lord, I am coming to a fuller understanding of that phrase from the Lord's Prayer, "Thy will be done." My unique meeting with Christ assured me that all that has happened to me was in the center of his will, and I am now able to believe with assurance Romans 8:28, "And we know that in all things God works for the good of those who love him, who have been called according to his purpose." I do love him, and I have loved him with all of my heart. Therefore, this stands true, and all the other circumstances that arise must be put in this perspective of love.

In my weakness and in my confusion that night in a motel in Wyoming, Jesus Christ reached down and ushered me into a new dimension of fellowship with him, "the fellowship of his suffering." In his love, Jesus heard my confused prayers and my unsure thoughts, and he understood my unique and desperate needs. I joined a great host of deeply suffering Christians whom Christ has met in their extremity, those people for whom there is no cure or miracle to make them whole again. Those who, like Humpty-Dumpty, cannot be fixed even by "all the King's horses and all the King's men." Those who must learn, with Paul the apostle, of Christ's sufficient grace.

I never really knew how many people are in this special fellowship because I only looked into the lives of the heroic from my wholeness. Now I have walked through that door and find a great crowd of loving, suffering, unsung heroes who are courageously living with Christ through the fellowship of his suffering. Paul went through this door and, though he sought healing, Christ answered, "My grace is sufficient . . . for my strength is made perfect in weakness." And Paul replied, "I will boast all the more gladly about my weaknesses, so that Christ's power may rest on me."

Since my illness, I have discovered a large group of deeply suffering Christians whom Christ has met in the same way he met me that night in the motel. Many Christians have found that when life completely tumbles in, when they are without strength or any hope or help for themselves, or when their minds become too tangled to even hold thoughts, that God overrules the circumstances and that Christ comes to minister to them at the very point of their need.

I will never again be able to preach or to teach. The only service I can do is listen and pray. However, even in my slight ability to do this, I have been so blessed by the calls of those who have experienced the "fellowship of his suffering." I have received calls from quadriplegics, from people in mental hospitals, from loved ones whose partners have lost their minds, from young people who blew their minds away with drugs, and from those who hurt as they have learned they have a terminal illness. We can pray and cry together and wonderfully identify with the person of Jesus our Savior who is reaching down to help us when life tumbles in.

Shortly after this experience of meeting Jesus Christ in such a wonderful and precious way, my health failed again, and we had to fly home to Miami so I could be hospitalized. However, this time it was different. This time I knew that Christ was with me, and I was determined to finish out my ministry with sermons explaining to my people how all of this could possibly be in the center of God's will. I love my congregation, and I love the people of Miami to whom we minister. I thought about my own predicament, and the thousands of people who had been praying for my healing. I was persuaded that, unless I could share my personal peace from Christ, they might think that their prayers were in vain and that perhaps God had failed. As I lay in the hospital, I resolved that I would ask my church officers for the opportunity to preach a series of five farewell sermons. I felt compelled to preach them regardless of my then stuttering speech and impaired vision. I prayed to God, "Please give me strength to conclude my ministry with praise to thee, and with the triumphant spirit that comes from having run the race and finished that one course that was set before me."

FIVE
THE JOY OF THE UNHOOKED YOKE

Deep within my heart I knew these would be my last sermons, even though as yet there was no medical diagnosis. The diagnosis came only after three of the sermons had been preached. However, in my heart after my spiritual encounter with Christ, I knew that this was to be the end of my pastoral ministry. Above all, I wanted Bob Davis and his problems to be relegated to the lowest place and Jesus Christ and his grace and power and joy lifted up so that people would praise God and see his goodness.

By this time, the disease had progressed to the point that I could not do research or carry great biblical themes in my mind. I just wanted to give my personal testimony to God's guidance, love, and care through the years.

Throughout my ministry I had shared little of my personal life but rather concentrated on biblical preaching. Now it was time to tell my story before stepping aside. I shared with the congregation some of the things written here about the hungers and drives, both physical and spiritual, that shaped me.

As I served in the pastorate over the past twenty-eight years, Betty and I have seen miracle after miracle occur. There is no thrill like committing one's life to the Lord with some small distrust in his wisdom, and seeing him multiply weakness into strength, like the boy who gave his lunch to Jesus and saw five thousand fed.

My true servanthood began when I answered his question, "What is in your hand?" And I said, "Nothing but my car, my beautiful Chrysler." And it was sealed at that sewer junction at Toccoa Falls when I said, "Lord Jesus, I do love you with all my heart. I will serve you regardless of whatever task you call me to do." The path of being Christ's obedient servant just happened to be for twenty-eight years in the gospel ministry.

My ordination into the ministry was a high point of my life. Present were all the ministers of the North Indiana Conference of the Methodist Church. It was a double service. One part was to honor the old saints of the Lord, who had spent their lives in the ministry and were now ready to retire. The other part was to ordain the young men like me, so that we could officially begin our gospel ministry. This was a grave and holy time. This was not taken lightly. The sanctuary there was just saturated with prayer.

We young ministers who were about to be ordained were waiting in a side room. We were addressed by a district superintendent whom I regarded as one of the most godly ministers I have ever known. He again emphasized the high calling into which we, as servants of Jesus Christ, were about to venture. He emphasized that we were about to be put in the highest position of trust on the face of the earth. This trust was placed upon us by the people before whom we spoke for God. This trust was also placed upon us by Christ himself, who placed directly into our hands the responsibility and the honor of proclaiming his gospel, his Word, and his will for mankind.

I remember the old district superintendent brushing a tear from his eyes as he said, "Yours is the task that has to be more true and trustworthy than a president's or a king's, because you will be representing the King of Kings." He then paused and said, "Let me give you the challenge that someone gave me many years ago on my ordination day. If you dare, and this is one of the most daring prayers you will ever pray: If you dare, ask God that he would strike you dead before you would do anything to dishonor Christ and the high calling of the gospel ministry that he is now placing upon you." With no little fear, I dared pray that prayer. I am, forgive me, a little bit proud and thankful to come to the end of this ministry in an honorable state.

As I shared my testimony and stories of the goodness of God and the joy I had following him all these years, I knew that my people had caught the joy and wonder that was in my heart. Yet, I knew there was one burning question that all those who know and love me were feeling. Why? Why must it end now? Why should our "shepherd" be taken from us? God, where is your "goodness" if you can stop a disease like this and you do nothing?

I am a pastor and have that unique thing called a pastor's heart. For twenty-eight years, Betty and I thought about what Christ would have us do, and what we could do for the spiritual life of the congregation we shepherded for Christ. A pastor's heart makes you think more of the care of your congregation than you think of your own care. Now I knew that it was time to close my ministry. As the pastor of my caring and praying church, I knew that I had to bring a closure to my ministry so that my people could understand the mystery of the sovereignty and goodness of God who holds time and life in his hands.

I wanted to answer again this question about human suffering, as I had many times before from the pulpit. Perhaps this time it would have more impact as I become a living object lesson, just as Jeremiah was to Israel.

Suffering is inherent in our world system since Adam and Eve broke faith with God. Absence of suffering will occur again only when all creation is in fellowship with God and living according to his laws. Even the created things are waiting for this reconciliation, as we read in Romans 8:22. As long as this fellowship is broken between God and his creation, suffering will occur and good people along with the evil people will fall under this curse.

Suffering will occur to many because of the circumstances and happenstance of birth. Certain ones are going to be sick and have some disease or another. Others are going to be at the wrong place at the wrong time and will have accidents. Many will suffer as a result of evil people hurting them, through no fault of their own. Some will suffer all their lives because of the wrong choices they have made.

The Bible tells us when a rainstorm sweeps across a field it does not pick its way just to drop its water on the holy and the nice people, but also falls on the fields of the unholy and the wicked people. God did not unbalance the working of nature in this way. For as Jesus said, God sends the rain on the just and the unjust (Matt. 5:45). Jesus said even more pointedly that Christians can expect suffering, persecution, abuses, and many other things just because they dare to stand for Christ. The world and Satan hate their Christian light and try to darken that light. The blood of martyrs stains the earth red in spots around the world where Christians paid with their lives for their stand for Christ.

God did not promise that when we became Christians we would be lifted above all of the natural troubles to which the rest of humanity is subjected. We are to expect our share of them: all the results of the suffering to which the rest of humanity is subjected, plus the persecution that might be the Christian's lot to endure for his Savior. I want to leave the message that God's healing power does not always remove physical suffering. God has ways beyond our comprehension, and sickness and pain are sometimes part of these ways. The important point is that God is able to heal physically. But whether or not he chooses to heal the physical body, he always heals the spirit of those who surrender to his will.

Through the years I have experienced many healings. Some were answered prayer along with medical intervention. Others have been miracles wholly apart from medical assistance. As a young boy, I had a severe kidney infection. This was in the 1940's, before antibiotics or penicillin were available. The doctor told my mother that I probably had less than two weeks to live, and that if I did survive I would be a cripple the rest of my life. The people at Silica Church held a special prayer meeting, and that night I was immediately and completely healed. In fact, I was healed so completely that there was no residual weakness. I was able to go on and lead a very active life in athletics and all sorts of other strenuous activities.

God's healing power was again manifest in a very special way after I graduated from seminary. I was serving my first church. For some reason, the pressure of pastoral work drove my blood pressure dangerously high. After trying various drugs and finding nothing to bring it down, the doctor said, "You have a choice. The pressure of the ministry is killing you. You can either leave the ministry, or I can personally guarantee that you will be dead before you are thirty-five. Don't be a fool. Get out of the ministry and save yourself."

Needless to say, this was shocking news. My daughter, Debby, who is now twenty-eight, was just born. I did not want to leave Betty a widow with a baby to take care of. I grew up with a widowed mother and I knew how tough it was. Despite this seeming roadblock, Betty and I both felt the ministry was God's will. It took a great deal of courage to say together, "Let's go for it. It is better to be a dead man doing God's will than a live man out of God's will. Let's just trust God and keep going!"

Over the years, I have had several other frightening experiences with things such as pulmonary embolism, kidney stones that blocked my kidneys, diabetes, dangerously high blood pressure, liver malfunctions, and heart problems. In many cases the physicians advised me to cut back or to choose another profession that would allow me to live less stressful and more regulated hours. Again, Betty and I considered every proposition and felt that if the Lord called me to the glorious work of his ministry, then he would heal me so that I could continue until I had finished my course. This was a family decision, shared not only by my wife, Betty, but also by our two daughters, Debby and Becky. I have walked through the valley of the shadow of death many times, but I was sure that God's healing power would sustain me until my work was finished.

As you read the Gospels, you realize that Jesus did not heal everyone. He had the power to, but yet he did not. Physical healing was not always the answer, even for the people who personally walked with Jesus.

The Apostle Paul apparently came down with a horrible eye disease common in the Mediterranean countries. It blurred eyesight, and made the eyes into running sores. Historians tell us that people were especially hideous from this disease because secretions ran from the infected eyes and attracted flies. Bible scholars tell us this was the disease that Paul had because in Galatians he comments with wonder on his handwriting, probably as a result of the disease. "See what large letters I use as I write to you with my own hand!" (Gal. 6:11). He probably meant letters like those made by a child or a visually impaired person.

Why would God allow this awful thing to happen to Paul? Why would the Christ he loved and served so valiantly not heal him? Paul answered these questions himself. "There was given me a thorn in my flesh, a messenger of Satan, to torment me. Three times I pleaded with the Lord to take it away from me. But he said to me, 'My grace is sufficient for you, for my power is made perfect in weakness.' Therefore I will boast all the more gladly about my weaknesses, so that Christ's power may rest on me" (2 Cor. 12:7-9).

Christ did not heal the Apostle Paul. Christ is under no obligation to heal every Christian. If healing does not come, what does come? God told the Apostle Paul, "My grace is sufficient for you, for my power is made perfect in weakness." We discover in weakness a new fountain of grace. This was what I discovered, and along with it an amazing supernatural peace.

Now I come to a new phase in my life. As the writer of Ecclesiastes said, "There is a time for everything, and a season for every activity under heaven: a time to be born, and a time to die, a time to plant and a time to uproot, a time to kill and a time to heal, a time to tear down and a time to build" (3:1-3). And at the conclusion of this long list, the writer said, "God has made everything beautiful in his time" (v. 11). He has also set eternity in the hearts of men. Yet they cannot fathom what God has done from beginning to end.

I hope you understand as I have shared myself with you that in my natural state I am nothing. I was helpless, but Christ saved me and gave me a new life and personality. God has blessed me beyond my wildest dreams and has answered so many prayers in my life. The Holy Spirit has given me gifts and power to do the thing I wanted to do most, to be a servant of the Lord Jesus Christ. God gave me blessings and length of life beyond what the best doctors predicted or I ever expected. He has led me and strengthened me. What a heartbroken man I would be today if I had broken my vow to burn out for Christ and had followed the advice of my friends to save myself. How bitter would be my tears crying, "Oh, God, to save myself for what?"

The most wonderful example I know of Christ's healing power in my life is that Christ healed Betty and me on the inside. He healed the brokenness and despair that filled our hearts and gave us an entirely new dimension of his peace that surpasses all understanding, deep inside. The Lord is our Shepherd and he tempers the wind to the shorn lamb. He knew the medical diagnosis that we would receive, and he gave us a new dimension from his wonderful peace, so that inside there is not despair, but instead peace and rest.

The peace of Christ is so wonderful, and it goes before us to prepare us for life's shocks and to fill us as we endure them. A friend comforted me with these words: "Remember, the bigger the hole, the greater the filling."

Christ answered my prayers for physical healing those times when my family needed me and the very existence of Old Cutler Church was so perilous. I praise him for that. And he miraculously gave me these precious years that were so beautiful. Christ is now answering my prayers by giving Betty and me his wonderful peace. I love him and have served him, and now I must learn to rest in his love, throw away my pride, open my heart and my hands, and let God and his servants serve me in my weakness. For one who has served others all his life, it is hard to relax and let people serve me.

You see, right now Betty and I have two options. We can either be bitter and groan and be miserable and curse God, or else we can thank God for what he has done, especially for giving us his great healing power when it was so critical in our lives. We want to be happy and enjoy life to its fullest and to grasp each day and to squeeze each drop of joy from it. We want to spread joy and peace, not bitterness and discontent. These just may be the greatest days of our lives. Christianity works. In the most helpless, hopeless, and extreme part of my life, Christ is here comforting and giving life meaning, even when all I have to look forward to in this life is becoming a mindless vegetable. The assurance that another life is coming full of perfection and the reconciliation of all God's creation gives hope. And incredible as it seems, there is great peace and joy in our hearts and our souls. My brain may be dying, but in my spirit Christ has healed me, and I can say with the songwriter, "It is well with my soul."

The final sermon was the unhooking of the yoke. This was in a sense a victory service, for God had set the finish line for the race that I was to run. For some the race is very long and for others very short. The distance is not so important as the faithfulness of the runner to finish his race.

August 2, 1987, marked the finish line for me in the pastoral ministry. It seemed appropriate to me to use the Apostle Paul's text: "For I am already being poured out like a drink offering, and the time has come for my departure. I have fought the good fight, I have finished the race, I have kept the faith" (2 Tim. 4:6-7).

Notice the word *departure* in verse 6. It comes from the Greek word *analysis,* which means an unloosing, as of an animal from the yoke of its plow or a boat from its mooring. Figuratively, it referred to Paul's departure from this life, letting go of worldly cares and toil.

Imagine an ox that has been working hard. He has been laboring as hard as he can from the bright rays of the morning sunrise through the burning heat of the noonday sun, until now when the sunset starts to paint the skies with its beautiful glow. The old ox has worked hard because it is planting time. The time for planting is limited if you are going to get the seed in on time. Now that old ox is exhausted, going on with sheer willpower, even stumbling a little bit as he finishes his last furrow. Finally, his master drives him up to the barn, pats his shoulder, and says, "You can quit now, friend. Take it easy and enjoy your rest. You have earned it."

So on August 2, I laid aside the yoke of the doctoral hood and the yoke of the pulpit robe. Like that tired old ox, I was unhooked from my yoke of joy, yet a burdensome yoke that I can no longer bear because of my sickness.

I do not cease to be God's "ox" or servant just because the yoke is removed. I will just be his servant in another way. I cannot lead now, but I will follow in whatever way I can.

As I knelt to be set apart by prayer on my ordination day, I prayed that a certain verse might be lived out in my life. I wanted to live it so that somehow it might be read at the conclusion of my ministry. It was these same words of the Apostle Paul, and I still pray it will be said about me. "I have fought the good fight. I have finished the race. I have kept the faith."

I have fought the good fight, and at times it has been a fight and a struggle. I have fought with church denominations, with church leaders, with wicked people, and sometimes with the very demons from Satan himself. I have fought, not because I like to fight, but because sometimes in upholding the cause of Christ it takes a courageous stand and tremendous fight. God made me able to do that. The external fights are one thing, but the internal, spiritual fights are another. There is always the fight over the temptation of whether a person is going to satisfy his burning personal desires or do Christ's will.

I have fought a good fight. What a joy it is to say wherever I was and whatever circumstances I was in, without ever slacking off for thirty-four years since I gave myself to Christ, I have fought a good fight.

I also have kept the faith. Faith is a singular word. Here it is used to describe the simple, pure truth of what we believe. The devil, all the forces of hell, wicked men, and false religions all stand against us to try to get us to twist, or compromise, or forget, or not emphasize the faith that the Bible tells us to contend for, the faith that once and for all was entrusted to the saints. Down through the years, I have encountered many people who have tried to persuade me to give up this faith. But yet I can testify that I met all these attractive compromises with the same will that Martin Luther had as he said, "Here I stand, I can do no other."

Finally, I can say, "I have finished the race." The greatest enemy that I had to face in my life is not one that you would guess. It is boredom. When I am bored, I generally get into trouble. As one of my high school teachers wrote about me, "When there is no excitement, he creates his own." God knew this was a part of my built-in, prewired personality. That is why he set out the unusual race course that he did for me.

Now this was all in God's plan for setting the distance of the race that I was to run. He has given me permission to take the heavy yoke off at this time, and to rest from my labors. This is one of the reasons for the peace that fills me at this moment.

As I stood there on the last day of my ministry, I must confess I did so with some disappointments. Jesus said, "If you have faith as small as a mustard seed, you can say to this mountain, 'Move from here to there,' and it will move." I sincerely wanted that kind of faith. But I have never moved any mountains. I would have liked to. Jesus also said, "You shall know the truth, and the truth will make you free." All of my life I have studied and traveled to be the fullest kind of truth-seeker. I dedicated all of my spare time to it. It is only as I became older that I realized the simple fact that when one knows Christ as his Savior, he comes into the halls of ultimate truth. Everything else that one learns is merely augmentation of that singular truth.

Jesus also said, "Be perfect, therefore, as your Father in heaven is perfect." In my heart of hearts I longed to reach that type of completeness. But in my conduct I failed, sometimes quite miserably. In spite of the disappointments and my failures to reach that high ideal, how thankful I am to report that I do stand in that perfection. It is not by my own works or by my own righteousness, but rather by the blood of Jesus Christ that took away all sins. By his grace, I can doubly relax and enjoy my sure and certain salvation. How wonderful it is to know that the key to the door of heaven is not marked, "Earned by Self-Righteousness," but it is instead marked, "Saved by Christ's Grace and Forgiveness."

I now stand and wait as I always have—as Christ's willing servant. There is no bitterness in my heart. How richly I am blessed!

Is there disappointment? Certainly! At times when my mind is sharp I am ready to take up the yoke and do great things for my Lord, but then a few hours later when my mind fogs, and I have to lie down to recover my thinking in the dark quiet of my room, I know that God was right to remove the yoke.

God has sent many comforters to me during this painful time of adjustment, but perhaps the most unusual came from the grave. As I was cleaning out some of the file drawers at church in preparation for my resignation, I happened to come across some old English literature notes from my days at Toccoa Falls College. The English teacher, Miss Landis, was one of the hardest teachers I ever had in my life. She regarded teaching as her special service for the Lord. One of her course requirements was that we keep a notebook of famous writings from English literature. She said that perhaps one day these would mean a great deal to us. As I glanced through that notebook so begrudgingly kept by me thirty-three years earlier, I came across Milton's well-known poem, "On His Blindness."

I read it and tears filled my eyes, and an explanation filled my heart. Miss Landis, that old spinster, that precise teacher who was so cold-hearted in her teaching of English literature, gave a gift to all her future missionaries and ministers. We did not appreciate it at the time, but in her wisdom she knew that many missionaries would return home from the field broken. Some of the ministers would have to leave their field of service. Milton in his agony would speak to us and answer the great questions we would face.

On His Blindness

When I consider how my light is spent
E're half my days, in this dark world and wide,
And that one Talent which is death to hide,
Lodg'd with me useless, though my Soul more bent
To serve therewith my Maker, and present
My true account, least He returning chide;
Doth God exact day-labour, light deny'd
I fondly ask; But patience to prevent
That murmur, soon replies, God doth not need
Either man's work or his own gifts; who best
Bear His milde yoak, they serve him best; his State
Is kingly. Thousands at his bidding speed
And post o're land and ocean without rest:
They also serve who only stand and waite.

How these words struck me! Is my God such a hard taskmaster that he demands service when it is impossible to perform service? Is my God so unloving that he would drive me on even when it is impossible for me to go? Am I willing to go back to the first principle and be God's obedient servant, even if it means only standing and waiting in the blackness? This poem caused me to reexamine my relationship with my heavenly Father and again yield myself to his will and his way. All things are under his control, and as much as it hurt to accept this, if God wanted me to continue in the gospel ministry, he could easily have kept this disease from attacking my brain. The result of this experience was not commitment to a blind resignation, but a recommitment to a loving Father who had called me, molded me, healed me, and empowered me for his service.

SIX
ALZHEIMER'S: DISEASE
OF THE DECADE
Researched by the Final
Care Giver (Betty)

We are located in Miami, Florida, where we have access to the Mount Sinai Hospital/University of Miami joint study on Alzheimer's Disease and Related Memory Disorders. The center provides diagnostic facilities and support groups for care givers to help them cope with the devastation that this disease brings to the family psychologically, physically, and financially. The center also provides workshops on a regular basis, which update the research news and help families to interpret fact from fiction in the press.

The first workshop I attended perhaps spared us from untold misery. Dr. Carl Eisdorfer told us very bluntly, "Don't let yourself get on the emotional roller coaster every time the press writes up a new breakthrough in research. We are many years from a cure. Nothing under trial today has any curative power. The things we are experimenting with are only 'palliative,' that is, they may alleviate some symptoms and allow a little better functioning of the patient. You people in this room who have a family member with diagnosed Alzheimer's disease will not see a cure in time to help them. Save yourself the pain of running around the country trying to get help. There is no cure. The best you can hope is that those of you who are in the experimental projects may help the next generation to have a cure."

He went on to tell us that medical science does not even know what causes Alzheimer's disease at this time (1987).

There are many diverse theories as to the cause of Alzheimer's disease. The three most widely held at this time are (1) premature aging of the brain, (2) the accumulation of chemical or other toxins in the brain, and (3) lack of essential chemicals, especially the neurotransmitters in the brain. Obviously, since neither Bob nor I is trained in medicine, this book is not intended as a medically definitive treatise on the disease. I would highly recommend that if you are a care giver to someone who has Alzheimer's disease or any of the related dementing illnesses or memory loss, that you read some of the excellent books on the market that explain ways to protect your patient physically and psychologically. Bob, in a later chapter, will share some of the unique ways of helping emotionally and spiritually. We have not found these needs addressed in the books we have read on the subject and this placed a burden on Bob that perhaps this was the last service he had to offer. He hopes that by sharing his pain others' needs can be better understood and helped.

The title of one of the classics on the subject of Alzheimer's disease gives the first clue as to the magnitude of the task of caring in its later stages. *The 36-Hour Day, A Family Guide to Caring for Persons With A.D., Related Dementing Illnesses, and Memory Loss Later in Life* by Nancy L. Mace and Peter V. Rabins, M.D. is available in paperback from Warner Brothers, P.O. Box 690, New York, NY 10019. This book covers everything from the definition of various dementia to a very detailed "how to" on various management problems: dealing with a confused person who refuses to give up his independence, eating, bathing, wandering, incontinence, and how to maintain your own well-being as a care giver.

If you are more curious about what is actually taking place in the brain, you will find the book *Dementia, A Practical Guide to Alzheimer's Disease and Related Illnesses* by Leonard L. Heston and June White, published by W. H. Freeman and Company, New York, most helpful. Both these books may be obtained through the national headquarters of Alzheimer's Disease and Related Diseases Association at 70 E. Lake St., Chicago, IL 60601-5997.

The unique phenomena in the brain that distinguishes Alzheimer's disease from other dementing diseases was first described by Alois Alzheimer, a German neurologist, in 1906. He discovered with an ordinary microscope that the brain tissue of certain demented patients contained an accumulation of abnormal fibers. These tangles of filaments were called neurofibrillary tangles.

In recent years, the more sophisticated electron microscope also shows groups of nerve endings that have degenerated, called plaques. The more of these neurofibrillary tangles and plaques present, the greater the degree of disturbance in intellectual function and memory. Obviously, this kind of diagnosis can only be made after death in an autopsy.

A brain biopsy will also confirm these but the procedure is considered too dangerous to use as a purely diagnostic tool in the United States. Since there is no known cure, a procedure this dangerous would be unwarranted to confirm as a mere point of curiosity. The diagnostic procedure consists of ruling out every other possible cause of the memory loss that might be treatable. In the later stages the degeneration can actually be seen by Magnetic Resonance Imaging (MRI).

In the earlier stages, there is not enough degeneration to show in this way but there is a technique that can determine the metabolic activity of the brain. This is seen by the Positron Emission Tomography (PET) procedure. By injecting a radioactive glucose material and reading the concentration of the radioactive material in the brain, a calculation can be made, using computer techniques that show which areas of the brain are metabolizing the glucose. Dead areas show no activity. It is believed that in Alzheimer's disease the dead areas will appear first in the parietal and temporal lobes. Since this procedure is still in the experimental phase, we cannot say for sure, but it has been in testing now for seven years, and it appears to be as accurate a tool as we have to date.

For many years, Alzheimer's disease was a diagnosis given only to the young who developed this dementia. Alzheimer's disease was synonymous to presenile dementia, and older adults were diagnosed with the term senile dementia. Recent studies in the last ten or fifteen years show no difference in the plaques and tangles of the presenile and senile dementia. Another recent discovery has piqued more interest in the genetic implications of the disease as we are now finding that all Down's syndrome patients show the senile plaques and tangles after thirty-five or forty years of age. Since Down's syndrome is carried on the twenty-first chromosome, perhaps there is a genetic link with Alzheimer's disease as well. Today we realize that Alzheimer's disease is no respecter of age, though only 15 percent of its victims will develop it before the age of sixty-five. It is interesting also that the earlier the disease is developed the more rapidly it progresses, giving strength to the theory that it is a premature aging process. One reasons then that the earlier it appears the faster this individual is aging.

Of further interest is the fact that in all brains examined past eighty years of age there is evidence of plaques and tangles, even though there have been no symptoms of dementia. Science has not yet determined what causes these plaques and tangles in the brain. It is clear they are not caused by hardening of the arteries, though a condition with similar symptoms called multiinfarct dementia is associated with hardening of the arteries.

There are no guidelines for predicting the speed of the progress of the disease but there are three recognized periods to the disease. The early or mild stage may last for two to four years with symptoms that often go unrecognized or are attributed to "We're all getting older." The major mental loss is memory for recent events and time disorientation. Because Bob's pastoral ministry demanded constant mental acuity and accuracy, with memory of names and details in his counseling and administrative duties, he became aware of his loss much earlier than many people.

Another symptom of the mild stage is lack of spontaneity. Bob noticed difficulty with creative thinking and also quick response which was often called for. I noticed it as a vague dullness, and since Bob is an insulin dependent diabetic, I chalked it up to low blood sugar. I'm sure he had a lot of unnecessary sweets and orange juice trying to clear the fog. I also thought that perhaps his hearing was failing due to the diabetes. I urged him on several occasions to have his hearing tested, but this just irritated him, and he assured me that he could hear as well as anyone. The problem was not his hearing but the fact that it took two or three times calling his name to break through the fog. Of course by the time it registered with him he responded with irritation because someone was "yelling" at him.

Now we both understand what was happening for the past two years. Now I take extra care to gain his attention without raising my voice. I may have to repeat myself without raising my voice and then wait for it to register. If this doesn't work, I may need to touch him to gain his attention.

Never begin speaking to Alzheimer's patients before you are absolutely sure you have their attention. If they catch the last few words of your sentence they do not have the ability to fill in the part they did not hear as we often do when we are healthy and this creates great confusion and irritation.

Depression and irritability are normal at this stage. This depression often clouds the diagnosis as depression can also cause the other symptoms by which we describe the early stages of Alzheimer's disease. The first time the irritability caused Bob to yell at one of his staff was very frightening to him. He has been a strong man who can keep his cool in the most trying circumstances, and this incident, which left everyone in the office trembling, caused greater distress to Bob than to the others. He voiced his fears to me, "Is this the result of the heart surgery? What is happening to me? My irritation gave rise to more anger than I knew resided within me. Am I losing my mind?"

The ability to see and read words silently and aloud is still retained. Even short articles of one or two paragraphs can be read with comprehension but comprehension diminishes in direct proportion to the length of the material. Bob finds after two to five pages into a book he has no idea what he is reading. The words are there, but the ability to connect them to logical progression and story line is gone. Writing ability diminishes but is still present, with spelling errors and words left out. The strangest thing is that when Bob tries to proof what he has written he cannot see where the words are left out in his handwriting, but if he types it into the computer, he can come back and fill in the missing words. It has been a great joy to discover this, so that the world of letter writing is again open to him.

Verbal expression is intact in the early stage but it may become too wordy. Also there will be errors in the exact word for best expression but it is not too noticeable in normal conversation. As Bob gave his five concluding sermons this past summer, these were certainly not with the flow of language he possessed prior to April, 1987. Mathematical skills were lost very early for Bob. Spatial relationships are impossible for him also. He cannot see how things fit together. If he is working on some little project around the house, he calls me to show him the order or the direction for fitting things together. When I lay them out for him he can complete the project.

The middle or moderate stage of Alzheimer's disease is the longest, often lasting ten years or more. It evidences increased and more noticeable memory loss. The remote memory begins to fade at this stage. Problems with orientation to place begin to develop. Bob has this symptom only on rare occasions and only in times of fatigue or when exposed to extreme amounts of visual stimulation. Having his glasses treated with #3 gray tint, which begins at the top and fades to a #1 at the bottom, has proven to be very helpful to reduce the reaction to bright light and flickering light. In fact, he is able to see comfortably inside the house and even finds this dark tint to improve his comfort while watching television.

I suppose this disorientation to place is the symptom that really made my heart know that we were dealing with Alzheimer's disease. My head knew all the best medical opinion had ruled out everything that they could think to rule out. The PET scan had shown the Alzheimer's disease pattern, the reduced glucose metabolism in the parietal and temporal lobes as contrasted to other causes of brain cell death that may occur in any of the other lobes.

The horrible truth finally gripped me in a motel in Bath, Maine. This was the trip in August 1987, following Bob's diagnosis and retirement, which we had intended to last for three months, driving leisurely through the United States and Canada. We started with a leg on the Auto-train from Florida to Virginia with a few days sightseeing in Washington, D.C. We meandered on up the Eastern Coast, hoping to reach Nova Scotia. Unfortunately, we had not taken into account the fact that New York City empties into Maine during August. I, unwisely, had chanced just a few miles more north of Boston only to learn there are no rooms after 4 P.M. At 9 P.M. in Bath, Maine, we learned there were no rooms within 250 miles. Right on the spot, we made a reservation for the following night.

Thank goodness for L. L. Bean in Freeport, Maine. We had wanted to visit the store anyway and they are open twenty-four hours a day with free coffee as well. The conclusion was that our car spent the night in L. L. Bean's parking lot and we took turns, with one of us perusing the store while one slept in the car. By noon the next day, when we checked into the motel, Bob was a zombie, despite the fact that he had had several hours sleep.

In the past, this sort of inconvenience would have been no big deal to either of us. Fifteen years ago, we had spent a month in Europe, riding the trains and getting an inexpensive overview by following tips from *Fodor's Europe on $25 a Day and a Eurail Pass*. Several nights we spent sitting up, sleeping on the train in order to budget some money for a Castle Tour or other extravagance. But this time we had gone over the edge.

As we carried our things into the motel room and I collapsed on the bed, thankful for a place to stretch my weary body, Bob just stood by the dresser. As I looked at him my heart was gripped by an icy terror. The look on his face was the one I had seen so often on his mother's face. How can I describe it? Empty, confused, blank, perplexed, unmoving. Yes, all of these. I said, "Honey, what's wrong?"

He replied in the most pitiful, childlike, pleading tone, "I can't find the bathroom." I went to him. "It's right here," I directed.

After two hours of sleep he was "back again." That look did not appear again until a week later after another too-long day of driving. We were already on our way home after only two weeks away. We had learned that we needed to learn some more about our limitations and also to travel at a less crowded time. This time the "look" occurred as he picked up the ice bucket and again stood glued to the floor. I asked, "What's wrong?"

He said, "I can't find the door." I showed it to him and he replied, "Oh, I thought that was the door to the adjoining room." Needless to say, I propped the door open so he could find it on his return from the ice machine, which was only three doors down the hall.

These two experiences taught me some valuable lessons. The one that is primary for any Alzheimer's disease patient: familiar places and routine experiences are essential for optimum functioning. Somehow we must balance this with Bob's need for intellectual stimulus, especially since he can't get this from books anymore. The second lesson was to learn where the fatigue limit is. Bob cannot be expected to recognize this and I, as care giver, must be very sensitive to his limits. I also must make them my limits, not his. I must say, "I'm tired, let's rest awhile," not, "Bob, this is getting to be too much for you."

In early Alzheimer's disease, patients, once they start something, are internally driven to complete it "yesterday." They lose the ability to break a task down into smaller units. They will keep on pushing to the point that they are stuck in a ditch, spinning wheels. This is true both physically and verbally. It is probably more noticeable in speech when they want to tell you something. They say it and then continue on and on and on. Also, if you try to interrupt their speech they will raise their voice and keep on going.

Impairment of remote memory begins to occur at the middle stage. Bob's remote memory can still be jogged by pictures and other mementos and, for the most part, it is intact. The annoying aspect is that rote memory is impaired even in level one, thus things he memorized are not dependably recalled. He may be able to give it logically in other words but to recite the Lord's Prayer or the Ten Commandments is virtually impossible.

In the middle stage, psychomotor agitation and pacing begin to be manifest, along with psychiatric manifestations. Bob does not exhibit all the symptoms of the middle stage yet, but he does have hallucinations occasionally, which so far he has been able to recognize as unreal. Even possessing this insight, his body still goes through the physical response to the unreal apparition with increased heart beat, profuse sweating, and an adrenaline rush. The horrible discomfort of this condition in which the mind "knows" it is being presented with an unreality, and yet having your body respond with no ability to control the flood of reactions, gives a feeling of being in "the twilight zone."

Fortunately, Bob has not exhibited any of the other middle stage symptoms, such as loss of abstract reasoning. Language losses become more noticeable during this period. It becomes more and more difficult to think of the right word for something. For instance, a patient told her nurse, "I like your wrong." The understanding nurse kindly guessed and pointed until they came to her ring upon which the patient delightedly said, "Yes, your ring." Handwriting deteriorates more, with grammatical errors joining the spelling errors of stage one. Errors are not noticed upon proof checking. At this stage the reading ability continues to deteriorate until eventually even a paragraph is too much to comprehend.

Social skills continue to deteriorate. Some people develop inappropriate sexual behavior. Clothing may be removed at inappropriate times or places or just the opposite may occur as the patient refuses to take off his clothes or shoes to go to bed. If the patient is taken to a store, he may shoplift something without even being aware that he has the item. A patient may cry to go home to his wife when in fact he is at home with his wife. Obviously, as the patient sinks more and more into the moonlight or drifts out to sea in the fog, only the very best and most caring of his friends will bother to spend time with him. His social skills can no longer carry an interest in the friend that could be considered to be mutually satisfying.

The third, last, and most severe stage fortunately lasts a shorter time, usually two years or less. This is the "nobody's home" stage, which Bob addresses in Chapter 9, "Death Before Death." At this point, communication skill is usually totally gone. Speech, if present, is babbling, repetitious, and incomprehensible. Comprehension appears to be highly impaired, or if there is comprehension, the patient has little ability to act upon it or let the speaker know that he has understood. Some care givers report that there is sometimes a look in the eye that makes them believe something has gotten through the fog.

The patient has no ability to care for even the most basic needs. He must be bathed, fed, dressed, and diapered. Truly, it is the final stage of man, when he reverts to infantile dependency. Walking becomes more and more difficult, with short shuffling steps or "sticking to the floor." This is a strange phenomenon in which the patient tries to move but the message just can't get through from the brain to the leg and foot as to how to pick it up.

Recognition of family and friends is sporadic and eventually non-existent. Bob's mother thought he was her brother Jess for the last six months of her life. She just couldn't understand why he looked so young because Jess, who had been dead for over ten years, was older than she was. When Bob answered that he was Bob, her son, she would become angry. We have since learned that it probably would have been better to have changed the subject or diverted her attention to something else. Logic and reason are rather useless techniques to use with the late middle stage and last stage of the disease.

Bowel and bladder incontinence, along with uncontrollable muscle jerks and repetitive motions and even seizures, may occur in this late stage. Along with this decreased motor tone come the secondary medical complications. Without careful supervision, malnutrition will also be a problem at this point as the patient may no longer experience hunger and thirst. He also may forget how to swallow. If you are feeding him, you must continue to tell him to swallow until he responds.

Every patient will not experience every symptom described here. Bob has some other symptoms, which we don't yet know if they are related to the Alzheimer's disease or something else. For instance, every time Bob is beginning to "lose it" mentally, he begins to cough. The cough continues to worsen until he removes all stimuli possible and lies down in a dark, quiet room. All the neurologists to whom we have spoken say they are puzzled by this, but we are plowing new ground. This is a relatively new field to be able to recognize the disease this early, and since every patient does not manifest all the symptoms that we do know about, there may be more markers than we have yet recognized.

SEVEN
THE ABNORMAL
CHANGES SO FAR

Some may ask, "What is it like to have Alzheimer's disease?"

Obviously the noticeable changes will be very individual according to the life-style and occupation of the person and the demands placed upon him. I know that many people were able to continue in their profession much longer than I. People who have a routine job that does not require mathematical skills or new learning may function at their job until they can no longer find their way to the work place.

Because of the particular demands of the pastoral ministry, I was made aware of my losses very early in the course of the disease. For more than a year, many of these losses were attributed to other causes, and I took every possible treatment to alleviate them. The trauma of surgery then brought considerable new demands on my body, and at this time all the measures to compensate no longer took up the slack. I had reached the point of no return. Life would never again be the same.

In my present condition (February 1988, just seven months since diagnosis) there are times when I feel normal. At other times I cannot follow what is going on around me; as the conversation whips too fast from person to person and before I have processed one comment, the thread has moved to another person or another topic, and I am left isolated from the action—alone in a crowd. If I press myself with greatest concentration to try to keep up, I feel as though something short circuits in my brain. At this point I become disoriented, have difficulty with my balance if I am standing, my speech becomes slow, or I cannot find the right words to express myself.

At my own speed and in keeping with my individual body rhythms, I can still act with the skills and knowledge I have acquired over the years. This book is an example of this. It was dictated at all hours of the day and night, whenever I had a clear enough mind to string thoughts together.

In my rational moments I am still me.

Alzheimer's disease is like a reverse aging process. Having drunk from the fountain of youth one is caught in the time tunnel without a stopping place at the height of beauty and strength. Cruelly, it whips us back to the place of infancy. First the memories go, then perceptions, feelings, knowledge, and, in the last stage, our ability to talk and take care of our most basic human needs. Thrusting us headlong into the seventh age of man, "without teeth, without sight, without everything."

At this stage, while I still have some control of thoughts and feelings, I must learn to take on the role of the infant in order to make use of whatever gifts are left to me.

A baby must have its own special environment to be safe and happy. It starts out in a crib, moves on to a playpen, and then goes into its own room and, after five or more years, is trusted outside the house with minimum supervision. The patient with Alzheimer's disease must move in the opposite direction from freedom. Someone must constantly monitor the amount of freedom and self-determination in order to keep the patient safe and able to function at top level.

Patients have to determine the size of their playpen. If they go outside the playpen in their normal life, then, like a baby, they are liable to be hurt, and they are certainly very vulnerable. All the books written on caring for Alzheimer's disease patients stress this point—to maximize the potential for living, the patient must remain in familiar surroundings and follow an established routine.

RITUAL

Now that I am developing a ritual with which I can be comfortable, I begin to see the great value of establishing a routine within my limits. It is easy now to understand the seemingly boring routines our parents got into in their later years. At the time we watched our parents do this we tried to bring more variety into their lives only to be met with rejection or scorn. They intuitively had been doing the very thing that science now tells us to establish in order to reduce confusion to a diminished brain capacity.

In the 1950's, my physiology and psychology textbooks taught that the brain does not get tired. They stated that only the physical functions of muscle fatigue, cramps, and eyestrain intrude on our attention span so that we have greater difficulty thinking. I do not know the proper medical description for what occurs, but I do know that the ability to function intellectually rises and falls with the amount of time I have been trying to concentrate and the amount of external stimuli to which I have been exposed. If I do not listen to my body and withdraw from the overstimulation, it takes several days for my intellectual abilities to return. This is very frightening because I can't help wondering each time this happens if I have pushed myself totally over the line of no return.

This past December we took our little family to Disney World. The rides with their blinking and flashing lights, the confusion of the crowds, the long waits in line, and particularly the special effects shows of Epcot totally exhausted my reserves. It became difficult to maintain my balance without something to steady me. I couldn't make a decision as to what I wanted to do. I needed to go to the room and lie down but I couldn't figure out what to do to relieve my discomfort. Finally, my speech became slow and my wife insisted that I be taken to the room. I lay in a dark room, listening to the tapes that keep my mind from falling into the "black hole" that tries to suck me in every time I stop concentrating on something. I spent six days lying in a dark room upon our return from Orlando. For a while I thought that I had lost everything but I began to recoup my ability to function, to leave the house alone, to visit with friends, to dictate portions of this book after more than two weeks of being a couch potato.

Leaving the routine of being around my familiar home, having more people and excitement around than I am accustomed to, varying my ritual for taking care of my grooming and health care, being unable to lie down and nap at my usual times, all brought me to a place of being unable to make even the most basic decisions for myself, of not even being aware of how to relieve my discomfort. This experience taught me that if I want to function at the top of my limited capacity, I must establish a routine and keep to it. I must stay away from crowds, blinking lights, too much emotional or mental stimulation, and must not become physically exhausted. I have to set the bounds of my playpen, even though it is annoying to give up the freedom of "hanging loose." I must seek out social contacts in groups of ten or less. I must avoid shopping centers and large athletic stadiums.

However, I can still go and work in the yard, I can enjoy church worship services and my friends there, and I can still go out in the midst of nature and enjoy places like the Everglades. The most important thing is finding out where I become the most lost and confused, and then staying away from those places so that I can enjoy life in my safe "playpen." Right now, I am very happy in my playpen, yet I realize that it will grow smaller and I will be compelled to adjust to this if I am to function at my highest level.

Two years ago, I was able to handle sudden surprising situations on a routine basis. Now I am completely paralyzed mentally if I am thrown a question that demands an immediate decision on my part. I must protect myself from being thrust into an unexpected situation. My wife answers the phone, or if she is gone I turn on the answering machine. This gives me a moment to assess who is calling and prepare myself to speak with them.

Betty and I have traveled extensively. We have visited more than thirty countries and almost all of the fifty states. Every vacation was a new experience in learning and relationships. I grew by new experiences. I am naturally adventuresome, and we enjoyed every new adventure possible. Those days are over forever. Because of my disease, the new and the strange have to be eliminated. Fear and tension fill me before any new event, even a wonderful event. I have to stay close to home and have less mental and emotional stimulation if I am going to have a more normal and peaceful life.

Along with the need for ritualism, I find that I am now a victim of obsessive behavior. Whatever I start, I want to get finished as soon as possible with no interruptions. An unfinished task preys on my mind until it is completely finished. This is the direct opposite of what I used to be. I used to read four or five books at a time and leave them turned down throughout the house so I could pick one up and read first one and then the other. I had a dozen projects going at the same time and could leave one and be refreshed by picking up the next one and working on it awhile. I was exhilarated by having dozens of balls bouncing in the air so that life did not become stale. Now I can only concentrate on one thing at a time and, much to everyone's distress, this thing occupies my mind and obsesses me until it is completed.

It is an old military maxim that the best generals win because they choose their battlefields carefully. The same thing is true with the early Alzheimer's patient. There are times when we cannot function and we need to withdraw and regroup. There are situations that we know we cannot handle. In spite of all the pushing and urging of friends and family who insist that we will have a wonderful time, the patient senses that it will lead to his mental devastation. There are times when the patient needs to be alone in order to keep everything in proper perspective, and the request to drop out of life or out of a situation at a particular time should be carefully considered.

At this point in my life I can still sense when I need to retreat from some situations, and my guess is that other patients have a better sense of what they should avoid than care givers may be willing to give them credit for knowing.

PARANOIA

Paranoia is another of the painful changes that has accompanied my journey into Alzheimer's disease. I was a strong, self-willed, self-disciplined man, and I thought that nothing could ever shake my mind. For years I have claimed Isaiah 26:3-4 as a promise for those who trust God. "You will keep in perfect peace him whose mind is steadfast, because he trusts in you. Trust in the Lord forever, for the Lord, the Lord, is the Rock eternal." I do trust the Lord completely, not just because of blind faith but also because God has proven himself to provide for my every need in every situation. Yet, the devastation wrought by this disease brought me to despair. Gradually, because of not hearing, not remembering, or not comprehending, fear swept over me as I lost more and more control of my circumstances. I was gripped by paranoia. The saddest part is that I became distrustful of those who loved me and had my best interest at heart.

I saw what was happening in me and I could name it at the time as paranoia. However, even though I saw it happening to me, I could do nothing to stop the feelings. I worried particularly about money. There was no reason to worry about money. The church took care of me wonderfully well as they made sure that my salary continued until our very adequate disability plan took effect. I cannot imagine the pain that it caused my friends, but I know that during this time I kept asking silly questions like "Is the insurance paid?" or other questions of this nature. I had such a great fear. I doubted any financial security. It was irrational, but I could do nothing to control the fear. After several months of constant reassurance from my friends and my wife, I am better able to deal with these paranoid feelings. If I start down the worry path about who or what is out to get me, my wife or daughter brings me back with a gentle reminder that, "Your paranoia is talking again."

Having experienced these feelings makes me wonder if this is the reason why people with dementia are found hoarding strange items. The loss of self, which I was experiencing, the helplessness to control this insidious thief who was little by little taking away my most valued possession, my mind, had made me especially wary of the rest of my possessions in an unreasonable way.

This paranoia that accompanies Alzheimer's makes me fearful of so many things and has completely changed my personality. Right now, I am able to recognize many of these things, but later on as the disease progresses I realize that it is going to be a burden to everyone. My goal now is to try to program myself to let Betty worry about the things that I cannot be reasonable about. I must make more conscious effort to trust God for the future. Each time I dignify the paranoia with an action based on the improper feeling, I strengthen the hold the paranoia has on me. Each time I face a paranoid fear and say, "I reject you and your hold on me for my trust is in the Lord and I will not fear what men can do to me," I have won the battle for my mind one more day.

FAILURES AND MISTAKES

Certainly one of the very real fears felt by anyone with early Alzheimer's disease is the fear of failure. I live with the imminent dread that one mistake in my daily life will mean another freedom will be taken from me. Each freedom taken places me in a smaller playpen with a tighter ritual to maintain myself.

For example, any housewife can forget a pan on the stove and burn dinner. She and her family just laugh about it and get a can of something else out for supper. If a person with Alzheimer's gets caught burning something, it is a severe tragedy, another marker of the progress of her incompetency for self-sufficiency. In all likelihood, it will take away forever her opportunity to cook unless she has a very understanding, loving family who will allow her to cook but will be willing to keep an eye on the stove without her knowing it. For the healthy person, this oversight will be just an honest mistake, but for the person with Alzheimer's, it may be the end to a whole line of productivity.

What fear this produces! The thought that one moment of inattention will change your life forever! I can still drive my car. So far my physical response time has not been greatly affected. My great problem is that of getting lost. Therefore, I limit my driving to a small radius around my home unless someone is with me to give directions. I also limit myself to driving only when I am well rested and feeling alert. However, I realize that in the old days I could easily have a fender bender in the Miami traffic and it would be no big deal. It happens all the time. Today if I have a fender bender, in all likelihood it will be the end of my driving career. Mistakes are not easily forgiven or forgotten. They often produce great loss of freedom and sense of person. I find myself becoming much more careful and timid, not from paranoia alone but as a result of these very real fears of failure.

DISORGANIZATION

It is very painful to go into crowds. When I sit in the middle of a large audience, I find myself becoming more and more panic-stricken, and quite often I will leave the church service, confused and completely drenched with sweat. I do not enjoy large crowds, and I can barely keep up with the people that I meet in the stream of people without becoming confused and having to sit down and regroup my thoughts.

In other places, such as shopping centers with uneven lighting and crowds of people moving in all directions at once, I become confused and completely lost. It is incredible that I can no longer find my way out of the center of a large shopping center, but my mind completely leaves me as I become totally disoriented. Even going into a large supermarket and looking at rows and rows of cans is mentally exhausting. When I do become exhausted, my walk becomes staggering. In a supermarket I can make it very well if I have a grocery cart to push around; or when walking in crowds I cling to the wall in order to give my hands something to touch to keep from going sideways. There is always the tendency in the confusion of a crowd to suddenly step sideways and perhaps to keep on going until I fall.

Headaches are a common occurrence. Whether they are caused by emotional disturbance or organic problems, I do not know. I do know that in times of emotional stress I have tremendous headaches that produce confusion and finally produce physical exhaustion. At the end, my mind blanks out, and I become unresponsive and uncommunicative. During the worst of these times, recovery does not come in an hour or two, but rather in a day or two. It is entirely different than being physically tired. Being mentally overworked takes a great deal of peace and quiet. I usually lie in my darkened bedroom, listening to tapes. Because I can no longer read, due to an organic disability, I am eligible for talking books for the blind, and these are great comfort to me at such times when my mind needs something to occupy it. This helps me in the middle of the night when I become sleepless and restless, and it helps me during the times when I have to withdraw in order to regather my mental abilities.

Waking up from sleep is a real experience. I have no idea where I am at times, and also I am totally lost. I have run into more objects in our bedroom and have more bruises from getting up and wandering around in the middle of the night than I care to state. Therefore, after I sit on the side of the bed to get myself orientated, I have to turn the light on in order to see. I am totally lost and forget the pattern of my own bedroom, even though it has been my bedroom for the last ten years.

At my worst times, I cannot bring myself out of this state of stupor. I need something to shock or stimulate me awake. I had a talk with one of my friends about making a battery-powered shocking device to try to bring me out of this quickly, but we decided against it as we did not know what the effects would be. One of my dear friends, Dr. Joe Davis, a psychologist who has helped me with this crisis, came up with a very simple solution. He said that if I would lay the roughest kind of indoor-outdoor carpet on my bedroom floor as a path between my bed and the bathroom, I could then follow the carpet with my bare feet, and probably the pain on my feet would rouse me from this state. It is an excellent suggestion, and one that should be considered. Again suggestions of this nature are hard to find because so little has been researched and written.

HEARING

My wife had been telling me to have my hearing checked for two years. I thought that I had a little trouble hearing on the phone at church so I had a special hard-of-hearing headset installed. As some close friends began to insinuate that perhaps I wasn't hearing everything, I began to check myself. I listened for the tick of the clock on the wall, and other little obscure sounds. When I concentrated I could hear perfectly well, so I inferred there was nothing wrong with my hearing. Yet my wife continued to speak loudly to me. I told her over and over again that there was no need to yell, as I could hear perfectly well. Strangely, she insisted that she did not raise her voice until the third repetition. I never heard her say anything three times.

Now it is clear why. I was missing many spoken clues. Whole sentences were passing by without my knowing it, and people could speak for my attention without my noticing. There was nothing the matter with my ears. The trouble was in my brain. I could not make the shift in attention until seconds or even moments after the intrusion. And on some occasions the intrusion never came to my conscious level. It was for this reason that I had to give up counseling, which I dearly love. I can still give wise and scriptural advice, but it is altogether possible that I would not hear the problem fully. Thus, I might give wise advice, but on the wrong subject.

PATTERNS AND PICTURES

I have lost my ability to fit patterns and pictures together. I find difficulty grouping things like I used to. A jigsaw puzzle is impossible for me. I cannot see how things fit. I cannot pack a car trunk. I can't figure out how to screw a nut on a bolt or how a piece of wood is supposed to fit into a slot. This ability to see spatial relationships is gone. I sometimes find the same difficulty relating verbal things as well. It is as if I hear things and they get into the wrong slots, which make no sense to me at all.

FORGETFULNESS

Memory loss is usually the first thing people think of when Alzheimer's disease is mentioned. I had always prided myself on my memory. I very seldom used notes during the day, nor even needed to carry a calendar for the day's appointments. About a year before my diagnosis, forgetfulness began to plague me. I found myself forgetting, not just obscure facts, but the most familiar things. When called upon to introduce the officers of my church whom I knew and loved intimately, I suddenly forgot their names or their wives' names. When called upon to remember the most obvious Bible verses, I would have it slip away. After missing one or two appointments, I began to carry a calendar and note my appointments. I even began carrying slips of paper to remind myself of certain things. Sometimes in teaching I would find myself grasping for the most familiar words.

Things learned in the past by rote were difficult to recall. I could explain the meaning of what I wanted to say but could not repeat verbatim. Recently learned material was more likely to be difficult to recall than things from the far past. With long-term memory, it is more like I have lost the access key to certain memories. Recognition is less impaired than recall. If a photo or a story jogs a past memory it will usually come forth intact.

PHYSICAL EXERCISE AND WANDERING

Wandering around and restlessness is one of the by-products of Alzheimer's disease. Many people have tried to guess why Alzheimer's disease patients are so restless and want to walk around at all hours of the day and night. I believe I may have a clue. When the darkness and emptiness fill my mind, it is totally terrifying. I cannot think my way out of it. It stays there, and sometimes images stay stuck in my mind. Thoughts increasingly haunt me. The only way that I can break this cycle is to move. Vigorous exercise to the point of exhaustion gets my mind out of the black hole. At first, it meant for me to go to a quiet room in our home and ride furiously on an exercise bicycle until I was panting and exhausted and my mind was clear. Now I try to schedule my daily routine with productive, physically demanding activity. Following this I rest quietly, listening to my tapes and sometimes fall asleep. When I wake, I am refreshed and usually more alert mentally. When I have had a particularly difficult night and awaken foggy and disoriented, I find that a stretch of vigorous activity helps me to clear my head.

ADAPTATION

My psychologist told me one evidence that I had been laboring under diminished capacity for some time before I was aware of the loss was the many compensatory techniques I was employing unknowingly. Some compensatory techniques are helping me maximize my potential. I must learn new ways to get things programmed into my brain, and I must find new ways to get my communication out to others. I must adapt to these handicaps for as long as I still have enough undamaged brain to do it. As noted earlier, tape-recorded books for the blind have filled the gap that my reading loss left.

A keyboard has taken up the slack that the writing loss left. Strangely, when I attempt to communicate in my own handwriting I leave words out, put down incomplete thoughts, and write in a scrawl, legible only to my wife. When I read over what I have done, it looks all right to me. I am unaware of the omitted words. Upon being made aware of the poor quality of my written letters, I thought I would try to type. Having been blessed with a secretary for the last twenty years, I had found no need to type.

I am not a touch typist anyway. In college we called my method the Columbus method: "Land on one key and then search for another." Much to my surprise, the thoughts appeared much more completely in the typewritten material. In addition to having less mistakes, it was easier for me to see any omissions. This track of adaptation led us on to a user-friendly computer with a word processing program. Now I am able to write letters and feel that I am not totally isolated from the world of intelligent people.

SLEEP

Sleeplessness has accompanied my journey into Alzheimer's disease. I feel as though I have forgotten how to fall asleep. I lay awake hour after hour every night. Sometimes I get only two or three hours of sleep. The less sleep I have, the more disturbed and confused I become. Depression, confusion, and paranoia accompany the sleep deprivation.

Before the surgery last spring, my mind held accurate photographs of all the places that I have traveled around the world. I could recall with vivid imagery the pleasant experiences I had in my life. I would turn my mind to this and to thoughts of prayer and thoughts of praise and slip off to sleep with great joy. Now with this diseased condition, when I let loose of my concentration my thoughts go into blackness. In this blackness, like the Bloom County cartoon strip, the terrible monsters from Milo's anxiety closet come out to haunt me. One night I spent hours facing down a tiger with bared fangs. Though my intellect knew this was only a figment of my mental pictures, my body reacted with all the adrenaline rush, perspiration, rapid breathing, and heart pounding of a real situation. And perhaps the worst part was that I could not move my body. I felt if only I could get up and start walking, reality would return. My body refused to respond to my will but rather responded to the unreal situation presented by my shorted-out brain.

I had to find a way to move from waking into sleep without getting caught in this never-never land of terror. I tried the usual radio talk shows and found them extremely distressing, because they were usually controversial subjects that got my mind whirling with the arguments raised. Music did not lull me to sleep.

As much as I hate to admit it, even the Bible on tape did not help. It rather awakened me as my mind would go back and pick up some familiar passage, think about it, think of when I had taught about it or preached on it, how it had been used, and then with all this stimulation sleep was gone. A relaxation tape made by my psychologist, Dr. Jack Tapp, gave me the first relief from this dilemma. His soft, persuasive voice talked me through the blackness to sleep. In fact, I used the tape for two weeks before I ever heard the end of it. But gradually even this lost its effect. If only I could find something else which was not stimulating to the imagination but was interesting enough to hold the concentration level out of the "black hole."

God answers our prayers in many interesting ways. A young couple, Phil and Debbie Rich, knowing I had lost my ability to read and wanting to comfort me, put their ingenuity to work and found some cassette tapes of Louis L'Amour. As unspiritual as this may seem, Louis L'Amour books of the American west have been favorites of mine for years. His word pictures had piqued my interest in the western scenery. I had used these books for years to turn off the whirl of my mind after late night committee meetings or counseling sessions. Again, I found myself turning on the same side of the tape for several nights before I finally heard it to the end. At last a way to help me past the "anxiety closet of my mind" and into the welcomed relief of sleep.

When I had finally heard all the tapes to the end, I went to the public library and learned that not only could I get regular commercial books on tape but that since Alzheimer's disease is an organic cause for being unable to read, the vast store of recorded books for the blind are available to me free of charge. They are available to anyone who cannot read for some physical reason, even to those who are physically impaired so that they cannot hold a book. Forms are needed from two doctors to verify the condition, and information on how to apply is available from most public libraries.

Since sleep comes to me so erratically now, I determined that during these times of wakefulness, which may come at two in the morning, I would not get up. I turn on the tape machine and listen to these books. I realize that if I allow myself to set a pattern of getting up to watch television or wander around the house I will disrupt the sleep patterns of everyone in the family. Therefore, I consider it a part of my self-discipline to keep my sleep confined to normal hours, and I lie quietly listening to a tape through an earplug or pillow speaker. I hope this will delay the time when I will create the "thirty-six-hour day" for my family with twenty-four-hour days of no beginning or end.

RESPONSES FROM OTHERS

I have been a public figure for twenty-nine years. When someone's profession thrusts him into the public eye whether as a preacher, a performer, or a professional athlete, it involves giving up certain freedoms of privacy.

We explained this to our children when they were growing up complaining about their goldfish bowl existence, telling them that "it goes with the territory." The easiest way to deal with the situation when people's lives are an open book is just to be sure there are no pages they would be ashamed for Jesus Christ to read. If our lives please him, there is no need to fear what anyone else may say about us.

Since my life has been open for public view, there was no way to hide what was happening to me. My ruling elders had been aware that I was trying to deal with an undiagnosed illness for more than a year. When I finally learned that there is no chance that I will ever be any better than I am now, I had no choice but to make it known and resign. For five months prior to my resignation, I had only been able to work in a very limited capacity. Being unable to carry out the duties of the minister of a large suburban church and being a limited human being are two vastly different roles. Not being able to handle the ministerial role did not mean that I immediately became a blithering idiot. Rather, it meant that I am now limited in my activities. I must choose my "battleground," so to speak. I need more rest and recuperative time after social contacts. I may not remember your name but if I have known you I still know you. The disease interferes with the access passageways especially to the names of things but I still know the thing. It is the vocabulary, not the concept, that is gone at this early stage.

As soon as my diagnosis was announced, some people became very uncomfortable around me. I realize that the shock and pain, especially to those who have a parent with this disease, are difficult to deal with at first. It was strange that in most cases I had to make the effort to seek out people who were avoiding me and look them in the eye and say, "I don't bite. I am still the same person. I just can't do my work anymore. I know that one of these days I will not be in here anymore, but for now, maybe for another year or two, I am still home in here and I need your friendship and acceptance."

Usually the response was one of great relief. Over and over the answer came, "I'm so glad you said that. I just didn't know what to say. I didn't know how to treat you. I didn't know if you could still laugh."

I am still human. I laugh at the ridiculous disease that steals the most obvious things from my thoughts and leaves me spouting some of the most obscure, irrelevant information when the right button is pushed. I want to participate in life to my utmost limit. The reduced capacity, however, leaves me barely able to take care of my basic living needs, and there is nothing left over for being a productive member of society. This leaves me in a terrible dilemma. When I go out into society I look whole. There is no wheelchair, no bandage, or missing part to remind people of my loss. It is difficult to meet the question, "What do you do?" When I answer, "I am a retired minister."

The next line hurts, "You look awfully young to be retired."

When you answer, "I have Alzheimer's disease," there is a strange look and uncomfortable silence. When Mayor Steve Clark and Commissioner Clare Oesterle, on behalf of the Board of Dade County Commissioners, presented me with a certificate of appreciation, this strange treatment was illustrated. Commission meetings are aired live on a cable channel and again in the evening for the benefit of those who are working during the day. That evening my family and I watched the presentation on television. During the shifting back to their seats, some of the commissioners, unaware that their microphones were open, were laughing and commenting, "He sure talks fine for someone with Alzheimer's."

For some reason some segments of society have a hard time dealing with a person who is just partly here. If you are unable to carry on all the responsibilities of your work, you should be bedfast or at least drooling on yourself.

One of the children at church illustrated this very well. After the final sermon and tearful farewell party and our very abbreviated trip, we returned to church to worship. This precious child of about eight years old, unhampered by the restrictions of manners, greeted me with his honest question, "Dr. Davis, why aren't you dead yet?" I gently explained, "The disease I have just kills your brain a little at a time, and I will probably be around for a while longer. I will worship here at the church even though I can't be the minister anymore."

As I have visited many nursing homes in my twenty-nine years of ministry, I have seen many people afflicted with one kind of dementia or another. When I relate to them, I do not do so with the assumption that they are silly, old, helpless people. I see the person they once were. If I did not know the person before the dementia, I tried to learn about them from a friend or relative. There is still a part of that vital person living inside that sometimes helpless-looking body, a person who deserves to be treated with dignity. Just because a person is incontinent or requires feeding does not give some eighteen-year-old twit the right to call them "dearie," or "sweetie."

Watching some of the Alzheimer's day care centers featured on television gives me the "willies." I could never bear to be talked to and treated like a child at summer camp. "All right boys and girls, let's all stretch our arms to the music; let's dance the hokey pokey."

I am repulsed by activity directors on cruise ships, much less some twenty-year-old trying to get me to play childish exercises to rock music. I'm sure I would try to get back to my room and if stopped in this attempt I would become churlish and belligerent. If the insensitive director continued to push or became condescending and began to pat my arm, I would probably explode with all the violence pent up in my six-foot-seven frame. If I were then restrained or tied in my chair, my fury would take me right out of my mind.

Why? Is this a result of Alzheimer's disease? No, this is how I would react now in my best state of mind. I cannot stand the beat of rock music or the bouncing around of even senior citizen aerobic exercise classes. Human dignity demands that I have the right of refusal for any activity or entertainment that I do not perceive as entertaining. I deserve the right to withdraw from any situation and to go to a place of quiet and calm that I have appreciated over the years.

As a caring professional minister, I have learned many things over the years. A person even in a comatose condition often hears what is said in the room. Relatives have been surprised on many occasions to learn that the comments they made in the presence of a comatose individual have been repeated to them when the patient regains consciousness. A person in whatever state of dementia deserves to be treated with all dignity and respect. In my twenty-nine years in the ministry, I have always called people by their title or Mr. or Mrs. until our friendship put us on a first name basis. I have never appreciated nurses and aides who greet me with over-familiarity.

When I called on persons suffering from any kind of mental loss, I let them tell me whatever was on their mind, and tell it as many times as they felt necessary. Then I tried to gently guide their thoughts back to an earlier, happier time. As they relaxed with their comforting memories, I then guided the conversation to the goodness of God and encouraged them to pray with me.

In Alzheimer's disease there is the loss of the personality, a diminished sense of self-worth. A highly productive person has to wonder why he is still alive and what purpose the Lord has in keeping him on this earth. As I struggle with the indignities that accompany daily living, I am losing my sense of humanity and self-worth. Blessed is the person who can take the Alzheimer's patient back to that happier time when they were worthwhile and allow them to see the situation in which they were of some use. I have a basket of letters from these angels of mercy who have written to remind me of a time that I shared God's strength with them and helped them. These have been my sustenance during these dark months of loss.

HOW ONE GOES INTO SOCIETY

I am not yet ready to be a hermit, even though there are times when I must insulate myself and regroup my diminishing resources. When I go into a large group of people, I know my friends, but the stimulus comes too quickly for my brain to sort out names. I smile and say hello to everyone. If I see someone approaching me, I try to ask the first question. It will be a timely question but one that makes little difference what the answer is. It may be as general as, "What do you think of the Miami Dolphins this year?" or "Isn't this weather incredible?" Sometimes this will buy me enough time to bring to mind some personal information so that I can ask about their work or family. This puts the burden of the first answer on them, and it allows me to sort things out and get them in their proper perspective. Blessed is that person who comes up to me and tells me his name first and reminds me of some experience we have shared. Usually this kind of approach on their part suddenly triggers a flow of memories that is almost impossible for me to recall by just reaching into the blankness.

Much of my life has been spent in the midst of large crowds of people. Now I find the maximum size group of people for me is no more than eight or ten. In larger groups I go into such overload that I have to withdraw and leave the group early. I still need social contact, but it must be limited to just a few people at a time and with little stimulation. Extraneous noise, such as a loud television set, a barking dog, or children who constantly interrupt and vie for attention produce overload so that I can no longer participate in the conversation. I develop a headache and begin to cough uncontrollably. The only remedy for this is a quiet, dark room.

LETTING GO RELEASE

As a pastor, I have been through many heart-breaking situations with parents who had a dementia of one kind or another. The difficulty they brought on themselves and their children because they refused to recognize their diminished capacity for good decision-making was tragic. I have seen them give away fortunes and do many other foolish things. I do not want this to happen to me.

I have given my wife the ability to make all decisions for the family. An attorney set up a durable power of attorney for her so that when I become totally incapacitated she will not have to resort to the courts for the authority to use our resources. She has the authority to make any legal decision on my behalf. I cannot function with any external pressure weighing on me. Since I can no longer do mathematical calculations, it would be foolish for me to hang on to the financial decision-making.

It is humiliating to give up our areas of responsibility. There is a distinct feeling of the loss of self and all that we have been. Yet all is not gone. I have chosen to give up those areas where I will be met with failure or my wife would be filled with aggravation at having to live with the consequences of my foolish decisions. It is better to release willingly those areas and concentrate on the areas where I still have some ability. Just as my wife gave up her right to self-determination when she married me and vowed to love, honor, and obey, so now in my weakness I willingly relinquish to the woman who has modeled the wife in Proverbs:

> A wife of noble character who can find? She is worth far more than rubies. Her husband has full confidence in her and lacks nothing of value. She brings him good, not harm, all the days of her life. (Prov. 21:10-12)

This act of relinquishing to her has relieved me of many of the things that would rob me of peace.

EIGHT
SPIRITUAL CHANGES THAT
BRING CONFUSION

What does it feel like to have Alzheimer's disease? I have already mentioned in a previous chapter the devastation of losing self-confidence, parts of the old independent personality, memory, pride as I became a care receiver instead of a care giver, and the ability to control some of my physical functions. The worst personal loss was the spiritual change that suddenly came to me. All these changes came in the matter of a few weeks. All these are permanent changes that happened to me, Bob Davis, who in the past was often described as a giant in the faith.

Perhaps the first spiritual change I noticed was fear. I have never really known fear before. At night when it is total blackness, these absurd fears come. The comforting memories can't be reached. The mind-sustaining Bible verses are gone. The old emotions are gone as new, uncontrolled, fearful emotions sweep in to replace them. The sweetness of prayer and the gentle comfort of the Holy Spirit are gone.

I am alone in the blackness. Suddenly, ridiculous, absurd fears creep into my mind. I know they are ridiculous and unreal, but they still come. Suddenly, in spite of my best efforts my mind becomes fixed upon these things—glued to them so strongly that I do not have the power to get my mind off these absurd, ridiculous, devastating, fearful things. I have become so frightened that I have drenched the bed with sweat. I personally discovered the full meaning of what the psalmist called "the terror by night" (Ps. 91:5). By faith I know the Lord is here to give me all the protection mentioned in this long-ago memorized psalm, but in the darkness and weakness of the night, my shattered emotions shout louder than my faith to my frightened spirit.

Sometimes these fears come even in the daylight as I am gripped in a trancelike state. In such a condition, people can even talk to me and I can grunt a response while those speaking to me have no idea what is happening inside me.

When I realize these fears are coming on, I have found that I have to physically move to break the spell. Often it is not enough to just move a part of my body, but I have to make my whole body move. I take a brisk shower, ride my exercise bike, or go for a walk. After such stimulation, the spell is broken, and I am saved from this internal torment. Since this works so well for me, I have to wonder if the ceaseless walking and wandering of Alzheimer's patients is their effort to raise themselves out of this agony of their own fears.

Neither prayer, nor Bible reading, nor meditation, nor assurances from friends, nor Christian radio, television, or tape programs bring any comfort in such a state. This is an organic physiological problem produced by the malfunctioning of the brain. How many afflicted Christians suffer not only from their unreal fears, but also the guilt of thinking that they have done something to grieve God's Holy Spirit or else they would be raised above this devastating mental anguish? How many Christians are loaded down with guilt by well-meaning children, friends, and care givers who sincerely feel that by their spiritual exhortations they can force Christ to penetrate into their loved one's troubled mind? All they are doing is unwittingly convincing them that they have perhaps somehow in their loss with reality committed the unpardonable sin, or else that they are truly cut off and forsaken by God. Like Job's comforters, misdirected friends unwittingly compound the afflicted person's perceived spiritual problem.

There is a way to help in these terror-filled times, but it is definitely not by reasoning with the patient. This is the time for comfort, reassurance, a soft touch, and a gentle voice with soothing words or even songs if you are so gifted. Whatever body language speaks peace in your family can be put to good use in this situation. As soon as my wife is aware that I am in one of these states, she embraces me and strokes me. She asks me to tell her about what was bothering me. As I talk about it, the panic subsides and I am made aware that I am in touch with reality again and that I am once more saved from the black hole.

Sometimes as I express my fears she reminds me of a Bible verse, and we praise God together for his goodness.

One of the first things that leaves is the appropriate emotional response. I feel both good and bad emotions at the wrong times. If the capacity for awareness is still left I can sense that the former emotional feelings are not dependable and trustworthy. However there is little or nothing that I am capable of doing to change my emotional feelings. I simply have to live through them and continually discount the effect they have on my judgment—if I can.

Our relationship to God is based, of course, on the fact of God's Word and he will not break his promise. He promised that all who come to him by faith in his son, Jesus Christ, will be made to inherit his kingdom along with Jesus. Jesus said, "Yet to all who received him, to those who believed in his name, he gave the right to become children of God—children born not of natural descent, nor of human decision or a husband's will, but born of God" (John 1:12-13).

My mind still can grasp this truth as I concentrate on it. I can claim this promise. I have confessed my sin and believed on the saving power of Jesus Christ; yet in the darkness of the night or times that I turn loose of the conscious concentration, I do not feel the Father's presence. The fellowship of the Holy Spirit is broken and random like a telephone connection where I talk but the messages coming from the other end are broken with static. Like the phone conversation in which one knows the other party can hear but their response is lost, it is not at all satisfying. I feel like an orphan child, alone, deserted, and never to be found again. I feel this way, but the mind that remains assures me on the basis of God's own word that he will never leave me nor forsake me.

I fear the day when my mind will lose this capacity as well. Then I must rely solely on those who love me to keep me close to the Father by their prayers, and to reassure me with songs and touch and simple words of Scripture. A friend of ours who had reached this stage beyond reason was fearful that she would forget how to pray. Each time I visited she wanted me to write the Lord's Prayer for her. Betty found a plaque with the Lord's Prayer in raised letters. I took this to her and prayed it with her as she ran her hands along the words. Using more than one sense helped her grasp the prayer and experience reassurance that she could still pray.

The private emotional relationship with the Lord that I enjoyed is distorted and does not comfort me now. When I pray, I often pray in silent blackness of spirit. Bible reading changes from being informative and informational into searching for passages that are inspirational and comforting. I am changing so that my old Bible study habits are disappearing. Now when I read the Bible, I often read the same short passage over and over again. Often this is a comforting psalm that tells about the sovereignty of God, a reading from the Gospels in which I am assured again that Jesus holds me as one of his special sheep, or a selection from the Epistles that tells of the majesty of Christ and how he helps believers through life, death, and eternity itself. These special passages become planks to be grasped in the emotional storms that sometimes threaten my basic faith.

In my emotional weakness, I lose the power to hold on or reach up to God the way I formerly could. The secret gentle whisperings of the voice of the Holy Spirit are stilled, or what is worse— distorted. I feel so cut off and alone from my dear friend Jesus. Before, I could reach up to touch him so easily or walk with him so naturally. If I did not understand what was happening organically in my brain to change these emotions, I would feel utterly lost and in the deepest of spiritual despair.

Over the years I have had to deal with dear, aged Christians with one form or another of dementia who have gone through such spiritual despair. I wish I had known how penetratingly they felt this internal blackness. I remember trying to shock them back to faith by rolling out a barrage of Bible verses and demanding if they still believed this. When in their confusion they agreed, I pronounced them cured by snapping, "See, it is like I told you. You believe, and God is faithful. You do not have a thing to worry about." How I wish I could go back to these dear old friends. Now I would put my arms around them, love them, tell them again the old story of Jesus, our good and faithful Savior and Shepherd. I would hold their hand and assure them anew as I prayed with them. How much strength I could have given them by reaching out and holding them! Now I more fully realize why we see the word, "touch," associated with Jesus so many times in the Gospels.

For instance, I remember the ninety-seven-year-old widow of an internationally famous Christian leader who used to sit in the corner of her room at the rest home and silently sob. She was sure that she somehow had committed the unpardonable sin. I remember clergymen of various stripes going in to try to convert her, to pass judgment on her by saying that she was trusting in her denomination or her good works instead of Christ alone, or preach to her by the hour. All of this was to no avail as she continued to sit grieving and crying.

If only I could go back and put my arms around her and hold her and love her. (Again I must affirm that touch is so important. For some reason people like us want to be touched or held. Maybe it is because we sense so many of our friends drawing back in our presence as though Alzheimer's were a communicable disease. Thus, perhaps we want to compensate by having people touch us, laugh with us, and treat us as they would a normal person—the normal person we still are at certain random times of the day or night.)

But what about this lonely, sorrowing old widow? This lovely woman had not lost her salvation. She had just lost her former ability to reach up to God and be fed by the Bible. She had lost the precious reverse side of prayer that comforts as she spoke to God, and God spoke to her. The old comforting Christian messages could no longer be absorbed by her troubled mind. I would love to go back and help her think back to her childhood. I would find out what simple songs and music she sang then and sing them again and again until in her confusion she finally grasped them. I would quote the old familiar twenty-third Psalm. I would hold her fingers and I would pull a finger for each word of the opening phrase, "The Lord is my Shepherd." I would emphasize that fourth word on finger number four so she could feel and thus further sense the word, "MY." I would tell her again how Jesus holds his lambs and assure her again that even though perhaps now she does not feel it as she once felt it, she is still one of Jesus' lambs and Jesus is still holding her even in her confusion, weakness, and helplessness of old age.

As I thought again of all of the people in the rest homes who are cut off because their mind is unable to comprehend all but the very simple and old things of the faith, I also thought of George Terrell, a bond salesman and a professional clown. This wonderful man in our church is in charge of our rest home ministry. Each week George goes to the rest homes to lead in the singing of these old hymns. He does more than just sing. He goes up to the faces of some of the withdrawn people and sings these old songs into their ears, takes their hands, and moves them with the rhythm of the music. Often when he does this he is rewarded by seeing that person wake up from his trance and smile or laugh. I know now that George knows the secret of how to bring the sunshine of Christ for one brief moment to their moonlit souls. How I wish I had known this secret in the years that I ministered to those older Christians who had passed from sunlight into moonlight!

In the closing days of my ministry, in which I was preaching some of the strong sermons of faith, I was at the same time internally going through some of this same spiritual anguish. I did have that burst of the supernatural peace of Christ that I referred to earlier, but there were hours of confusion when this left me. For the first time in my life, I knew the meaning of the words "darkness," "forsaken," "alone," "fearful," and "doubt." At times I was, as Paul put it, "of all men most miserable." Only because God left me with enough comprehension to realize that my feelings were the result of the organic malfunctioning of my brain, and that they had absolutely nothing to do with my spiritual relationship with Christ, was I able to go on. I realized for the first time that here was a reversal in my relationship to Christ. Instead of storming heaven with my thoughts, Bible readings, faith, meditations, praise, and enthusiastic exultations, I was too weak to even lift my eyes. I was too confused to do any of these things that previously had so characterized my Christian experience and ministry.

Thus this strong Christian leader was at times confused and defeated. To me in my rational hours this was absurdity at its highest. In my hours of despair I wondered what the solution was. It was only by great effort that I was able to begin to reverse all my lifelong thinking processes. I now realize that instead of holding on to God and pulling myself up by my exuberant faith, I have to relax and have the simplest childlike faith and let Jesus hold me.

All of this was inconceivable to me and totally incomprehensible to my friends who knew me so well over the years. One dear couple who were new Christians were able to see through me and read my confused heart. Mike Melcher is in charge of our sound system, and his wife Sarah works with the mentally handicapped children of our church. Perhaps because of Sarah's ministry, they were able to see some of these same traits in me. One Sunday they brought a beautifully wrapped gift to me. When I opened it I found it was a picture of Jesus. His nail-scarred hands were holding up and snuggling a lamb. Jesus snuggled this lamb so close to him that his face was buried in the lamb's neck. On the lamb's face was a look of pure joy and contentment.

This picture changed my whole spiritual outlook. I wept and cried out, "O Jesus, I have followed you as fast and furiously as I could through every path of life. Now I cannot! As much as I want to, I cannot. Now pick me up and snuggle me close to you, and help me to relax so I can enjoy this new relationship." Jesus did! This was another spiritual step of release that took place in my life so that I could live as a Christian with Alzheimer's disease.

I go to the services to worship God, but I cannot sing. I cannot join in the readings or prayers because my mind cannot do two things at once. Singing and group readings take several processes going on at once to listen to the others and pace my reading in time with theirs. Such a simple thing! But impossible for me now.

Suddenly I stand out in the worship service, silent and continually confused during the time of hymn singing. I feel that my fellow worshipers are looking at me askance, wondering why I do not join in. My newfound paranoia also sets in, making me wonder if they think by my silence I am showing disapproval of the hymn, the church, the musicians, or the people around me. This time of joy has been changed into a time of frustration and anxiety.

Now I would like to come into the service late, after the singing of the first hymns or any responsive reading. However, out of propriety I do not. How I long to again sing my heart out and thus fully express my joy, but I cannot. The sorrow of this and this sense of loss fills me so much that often tears come to my eyes—tears that only compound my paranoia and my ever-present fears of what people are thinking.

It was during this time of aggravation that I realized that by enduring this inner agony I was doing one of the braver things I have ever done. I stayed at the place where people knew me so well from my better days. The easiest thing in the world would be for me to move away into another area of the country, or run away to another church where no one knew me or had any expectations from me. Thinking back on this, I thank God for all the stroke victims, all those with Alzheimer's, and all those who suffered great physical and mental changes who stuck it out in their old church.

Before I had Alzheimer's, I thought that to these sufferers, their old familiar church would be the greatest place of ease and comfort in the world. Now I realize the constant strain of adjusting from the persons they once were to the person they have become is painful. I understand how hard it must have been on them to keep coming back to answer the same questions over and over again. I know how hard it is to deal with all the people who simply cannot handle being around someone who is mentally and emotionally impaired.

I understand their difficulty in saying no to the requests of some of their best friends who refuse to recognize that there is anything the matter with them. I understand when people make requests of them that in their heart they know they would mentally or emotionally shatter before they could fulfill them. They say no with such regret and such fear because they realize every "no" answer will keep them from being asked later to participate in something that they could do and would enjoy. How tempting it is to run and hide in anonymity! These handicapped people stuck it out, not because they needed us, but because we who were whole needed them to teach us of their new dimensions of true spirituality that Jesus had given them in their suffering. In spite of all that I have said, how awful it would be to lose our loving, caring church family!

I can no longer be spiritually fed by sermons. I can get the first point of the sermon and then I am lost. The rest of it sends my mind whirling in a jumble of twisted unconnected ideas. On the way home, I ask Betty to explain why this or that was included in the message. This way I get a little thought for the day as Betty breaks it down into digestible pieces for me. A Bible class causes disintegration from the strain of deep concentration. Coughing, headache, and great discomfort have attended my attempts to be fed in all the ways I am accustomed to meeting God through his Word. Must I be cut off?! How did people meet God before there were books? Thank God he will always have a witness to himself! Where do I find him? King David pointed the way.

The heavens declare the glory of God; the skies proclaim the work of his hands. Day after day they pour forth speech; night after night they display knowledge. There is no speech or language where their voice is not heard. Their voice goes out into all the earth, their words to the ends of the world. (Ps. 19:1-4)

Truly I am finding joy in God's creation. It speaks to me of my heavenly Father who cares for the birds of the air and the flowers of the field. Believe it or not I am comforted even by watching *National Geographic* television shows. As I see the intricately tuned balance of nature with a place for each creature great and small I am reassured that God still knows my name even if I can't hear him in the ways I once did.

Sometimes I can listen to the Bible on tapes. I find it less confusing to me to have a familiar voice reading it to me. Last year my wife recorded the New Testament to play to our grandson Bobby. So these are now a great comfort to me in my nights of nameless, dreadful fears. As I have enjoyed these tapes, I thought again of how I would change my ministry to the elderly and especially to any with dementia. I would do what ministers of bygone years used to do. I would read several comforting chapters from the Bible to them, slowly and clearly. Instead of taking sermon tapes, I would take tapes of my readings of the great chapters of the Bible.

Perhaps if you have loved ones whose reading is impaired you could make tapes of their favorite Bible portions, Christian poems, or old hymns. Thus at their time of need God can use your familiar voice to bless and comfort them with God's words.

Sometimes even these tapes are too much for my brain to absorb. Some thought triggers a flood of nonessential trains of thought that lead me off into less and less relevant ideas so that the real message is lost and my mind whirls away into useless activity. When all else fails, the "Promise Box" saves the day. These are boxes of cards with a Bible verse for each day of the year. Each morning I take out one of these and read it several times. I try to program this one thought into my head. I leave it lying out on the desk so that each time I go by I can feed my mind with this one thought from God's Word.

For the past ten years, I have preached, taught, and studied from the New International Version of the Bible. It became my Bible. Suddenly in my illness an amazing thing happened. As I struggled to read (and reading is now a tremendous struggle to me), I suddenly realized that this version of the Bible did not speak to my heart anymore. I then rummaged through the few books I kept after my retirement and found my old King James Version of the Bible. As I read this old Bible, suddenly the clouds began to lift. My mind somehow went back to the earlier years, and these old words from the King James Version suddenly began to fall in place and to bring new blessings. All my past ten years with the New International Version have disappeared, and now it is the old King James Version that speaks to me.

As I realized this, I thought of all the older people that I had hoped to comfort by giving them a much more readable New International Version or even the simple *Good News for Modern Man* version or the paraphrased *Living Bible*. I now realize my mistake. These modern words did not sound like the Bible to them. As their minds went back in time, they could not identify with these new words. They needed the old Bibles. I also realize now that if a person grew up reading and worshiping in a language other than English, he probably needs a Bible written in the language of his youth for his personal devotions.

An additional abrupt change was my appreciation of music. My church was well known for having the best in modern church music. With the six hundred people in our choirs and orchestras, we pioneered many modern musicals and cantatas. We always had the best in modern scriptural music. I thoroughly enjoyed such music.

Now suddenly I am distracted by this music. I disliked hearing it on Christian radio stations. I tolerate it now as I sit in the worship service of my church simply because of the joy that it brings to the musicians and the rest of the congregation. Amazingly, in just a few months what was before the most beautiful music in the world is now irritating music in which my mind cannot relate to the melody nor can it catch the words. Thus I am cut off from the music that I so loved and which had inspired me. Because of this new flawed musical perception, Christian radio gets on my nerves, and most of the music on Christian television somehow comes across like rasping performers on second-rate secular review shows. Because of the loss in the "switching station" in my brain, my mind can no longer automatically sort things so as to place them in the proper perspective, even simple things like sounds. Whatever reaches my ears with the loudest noise is that which penetrates into my consciousness and rules my perceptions. Thus modern music with its heavy beat produced by guitar, drums, or other dominating instrument is heard by me only as the beat, accompanied by mingled other sounds. A few minutes of listening to the beat of drums is enough to produce discomfort, even headaches.

God did not leave me comfortless in my need for music to fill my soul. One day when I was sorting through my record collection in that discard process that always comes at the end of a career or the end of life, I found an old George Beverly Shea record. It was one of the first so-called "long play" (33 rpm) records. Out of curiosity I put it on my phonograph. From that old scratched record came Bev's deep voice singing simple old hymns. I sat back listening, and then realized I actually was enjoying it. This music spoke to me. Eagerly, I picked out some of the old records with more old hymns. There came a sense of peace and enjoyment as I listened to these records that I had put away years ago as being merely historical curiosities. Somehow in the strange thinking of my mind I had reverted back so that new music was irrelevant, but the old music was spiritually refreshing. I again have music to bless my soul. Perhaps other Christians with Alzheimer's disease or other older Christians will have the same reaction.

As I listen to Christian radio, I realize they often have the annoying habit of mixing their programming. In the middle of some spiritually enriching soothing programming, they will slip an angry anti-abortionist or other such social activist whose tone is jarring to my emotionally sensitive nerves. Wanting my emotions to be protected (for if disturbed, my hard to control positive emotions can remain disturbed for hours), I switch off Christian radio and much of Christian television. The pure simple blessings of the Bible are such a comfort to me that I do not want to be robbed of these simple blessings and simple faith by anyone with a more complicated, strident message.

A journey into Alzheimer's is also a journey into the very basic simplicities in life. Perhaps it is because I know that my entrance into the glories of heaven is now so close that I feel the trivialities and divisions on earth are so meaningless or—if harped on—even irritating.

To have Alzheimer's disease is to suffer constant and often degenerative changes. There is nothing that can be done to stop these changes. No one knows how quickly these changes will occur. It is expected that they will occur much more rapidly for me as they usually advance more rapidly in a younger person than in those over sixty years old. As for the spiritual changes that affect a Christian, this is not meant to be a definitive or final word. All I can do is record the changes that I have personally observed at this stage of my illness. Hopefully, even these observed changes will open new windows that will allow loved ones to glance into the confused minds of my fellow sufferers. In my life I can only guess that I will lose even more emotional and mental control as these things will worsen.

It is my prayer that somehow God will hold me so that even in my uncommunicative silence Christ will somehow cuddle me close to him. I beg him for this in my secret prayers. With desperation I pray that I will not fall over the edge into that dark chasm of total blackness either psychologically, emotionally, or spiritually.

This journey into total complete blackness is a journey that I hope I never have to take and a misery I hope that I will never have to endure. But who knows? I cannot bear the strain of even contemplating it. All I can do is put it out of my mind as I absolutely trust in the love of my care giver, Betty, and in the unfathomable love of our magnificent Lord. My glimmer of hope comes as I realize that these glorious words of that old hymn, "The Love of God," were found written on the wall of a mental hospital.

> Could we with ink the ocean fill,
> And were the skies of parchment made,
> Were every stalk on earth a quill,
> And every man a scribe by trade,
> To write the love of God above
> Would drain the ocean dry.
> Nor could the scroll contain the whole,
> Though stretched from sky to sky.

Perhaps the journey that takes me away from reality into the blackness of that place of the blank, emotionless, unmoving Alzheimer's stare is in reality a journey into the richest depths of God's love that few have experienced on earth. Who can know what goes on deep inside a person who is so withdrawn? At that time, I will be unable to give you a clue, but perhaps we can talk about it later in the timeless joy of heaven. On second thought, all these heartaches won't really matter over there, will they?

NINE
DEATH BEFORE DEATH

If someone were to ask me what was the first great surprise I had in the ministry, I would have to say, "John Durbin."

What a thrill my first church was! At last the seven years of preparation in college and seminary were put into action as I finally had my own church.

My first ministry was in a little Methodist Church in Williamsburg, Indiana, a tiny farm village with one traffic light. I entered into the work of a pastor with enthusiasm and gusto. Life was exciting and wonderful.

It was perhaps two weeks before some of the members of my congregation asked, "Have you been to see John Durbin yet?"

I replied, "Who is John Durbin?"

I learned that he was one of the church members who had been paralyzed by a stroke seven years earlier. For seven years he had lain immobile in the bedroom of his home, unable to communicate except by giving grunting sounds.

In spite of my training in the hospital chaplaincy course in seminary, I, like most young ministers, did not like calling on shut-ins. After working up my courage for nearly a week, I at last called on John Durbin.

I had no idea how to communicate with someone like him so I

read a couple of psalms and closed with a prayer that God would heal him. John's response was two grunts.

In a small church you do not neglect anyone, especially shut-ins. Soon I made weekly visits to see John Durbin, and I learned his secret of conversation. You talked and made many of your statements into questions, and John replied by giving one grunt for yes and two grunts for no.

One day when I went to see John he cut off my trite remarks by grunting no. I started to leave, but he again loudly grunted no. I then asked if he wanted to talk about something special, and he relaxed as he grunted yes.

What followed was an elongated version of twenty questions as I threw out topics and he grunted either yes or no to guide me. As you can imagine, this was a long session—a session so jarring that almost made me stumble out the door as I left the room. What John told me that so shook me was "I want to die."

I was young and full of life. The thought of anyone really wanting to die had never fully crossed my mind. All I had ever seen was the bright rays of the rising sun that joyfully illuminated greater and greater mountains to conquer. Death—I was certainly not afraid of it since my relationship with Christ was so sure; however, I could never conceive of myself or anyone else desiring death.

Strange as it seems, these troubling thoughts took two or three weeks of contemplation before my mind could fully grasp that there are times when death is actually better than life. I had never really given it much thought. Yet as I thought of John Durbin lying in that position for seven years, I began to grasp how he could pray to be set free to run and leap in the glories of heaven.

This shaking personal experience changed my active theology. From this time on, my working theology took on the proper perspective. This earth is temporary, fleeting, and at times unjust and painful. Heaven is our real destiny. The only way life on earth can ever make sense is when we lift our eyes beyond the attractive bright rays of the rising sun on earth and see beyond the horizon the even brighter rays that emanate from the Son of God seated in glory in heaven. What a difference this vision has made to sustain my joy and enthusiasm on my earthly journey!

After I got over the shock of realizing that, for the Christian, in some cases death is even more desirable than physical life, I soon learned in the course of my pastoral work that many other Christians in extreme situations had also discovered this truth. Such lessons are not learned from theology courses or from religious books. They are not debate points to be argued over in seminars on death and dying. They are learned instead as we share and suffer with other Christians. I learned it from that kindly old grandfather who watched his wife writhe in pain from the inoperable cancer that was driving her out of her mind. With tears streaming down his face he said, "Elizabeth has suffered enough. Pray that the Lord will release her from this suffering and take her home to himself in heaven."

I learned it from the farmer's wife whose husband had suffered a massive head injury and now was locked in a crippling coma. With grieving voice she said, "May God forgive me if I am wrong, but I believe that this request is from him. It is certainly not from me. Pray that Jesus will take Jim home. Jim is such a man's man that he would never want to stay on this earth as a partially conscious vegetable. As much as I don't want to let him go, I know that Jim would want that new mind and new body his Lord has prepared for him in heaven."

I learned it from all the relatives standing outside that stark intensive care room where a vigorous twenty-year old, mangled in a car accident, lay stretched out. Not only his EKG but his EEG had now flattened. With one accord they stopped me before I prayed as they said, "Dr. Davis, we feel from the Lord that it is now time to change our prayers. Perhaps you had better stop praying for God to heal Bill. It is time to pray that God will take him gently home to heaven so that he may enjoy all the benefits that Jesus his Savior has for him there."

The non-Christian world cannot understand these feelings, since they have nothing beyond the grave. Thus they will fight at any cost to keep the physical shell of the body alive. That is why I insist on a doctor who understands our attitude toward life and death attending to me and my family. That is why long ago before anything ever happened, we all made out legal documents saying that should we be reduced to helpless vegetables with no hope of life that someone should pull the plug on the machines that were artificially keeping our bodies alive so that we may die naturally and be promoted to our eternal home in heaven.

Alzheimer's, like life itself, is terminal. Many doctors cannot accept the idea that Christians are assured of life after death. Their scientific approach to life refuses to admit there is anything beyond the physical life on this earth. As part of my clinical work-up, specialists wanted to examine my feelings about this illness and my coming death, with this as their frame of reference. When I was asked about my illness, I replied that there was at first total confusion, then a feeling of devastation as if an atomic bomb had been dropped to destroy my whole world. But then Jesus came to me in a special way to give the greatest peace and comfort I have ever known.

The doctor snapped back at this statement with a sharp retort to this effect, "Get real. Tell the truth of how you really feel. Stop denying it with this spiritual stuff."

After I assured her that these were the real feelings that changed my whole attitude she curtly asked, "Well, how do you feel about dying?"

I replied that when I received Jesus as my Savior many years ago all fear of death and dying were removed. Since I believe in and look forward to the second coming of Christ, I have for many years prayed, "Maranatha—come quickly, Lord Jesus." Thus I have lived every day as if it were my last—either by death or even more probably by the return of Jesus my Savior to take me personally unto himself.

This answer infuriated her. She almost shouted as she said, "How can you live in such denial?"

"But it is true," I said. "This has been, and this is my faith and my life."

"I didn't come here to listen to a sermon," she said as she got up to leave the room. I can only look back at this scene with a wee bit of humor. However, I am still able to sort out things like this in the working area of my mind. I had to think again of the more helpless Christians with Alzheimer's and realize how an experience like this would completely shake them and perhaps even rob them of what faith and peace their troubled emotions let them still enjoy.

Care givers, watch those Christians that you care for lest Satan inadvertently slip in somewhere to rob them of that last great secret resource—their deep emotional faith and peace. Particularly because of their weakened mental and emotional condition, their faith must be guarded and bolstered. Most other physical things of life make little real difference to them, but these spiritual resources are essential to comfort them in their final days of life.

The Easter message is the most glorious message of the church. Christ conquered death. Because he lives, we shall live also. This is our hope and our ultimate confidence. Doctors, lawyers, and theologians have debated for years at what point death comes. I believe that the death of the real individual sometimes comes even before his physical death comes. In my case, when the time comes that all purpose for living on earth is done, I pray that my physical death will then come quickly. I do not want my six-foot-seven frame, which was so eagerly sought after by professional football teams, to be knotted up in a static fetal position and covered by oozing bed sores as it suffers for the rest of its mindless existence in a remote corner of an expensive nursing home.

I do not want this mind that so served my Lord to torture me and do hideous things to me as Alzheimer's kills all that is truly me while it turns the rest of my brain to mush.

I do not want these lips that preached Christ at every opportunity for over three decades to be turned by the ravages of Alzheimer's into tools that babble obscenities and cursings—a curious symptom that overtakes many Alzheimer's patients.

Thus, in one of my final sermons when I told my congregation that I have Alzheimer's disease, I further shocked them with this unusual prayer request. "Please remember who I was. How well I can remember the deep pain I went through with my mother in her last years. There came a day when I realized, 'Mother's gone. She doesn't live in her body anymore. Just the shell of her eighty-seven-year-old body is here with us.' There will come a time when I can no longer function. And at that time, please remember the same thing. Bob Davis doesn't live inside anymore. Just his body is here. Bob Davis is the guy who inside was so tender and loved Jesus so much. He is the real person you knew.

"Finally when I get to that stage when my mind is gone—and research says that this will happen much more quickly with younger Alzheimer's patients than with older ones—pray that the Lord will take me home quickly. I have always believed what I preach and you have heard me preach of the wonders and glories of heaven. Why should I have to stay mindless on this earth when I could be enjoying all the glories of heaven? When I get to that stage of mindlessness, pray that the Lord will take me home to heaven where I will have a new mind, a new body, and such glory being with Jesus that it will just make you gasp for joy. Heaven is what life is all about! In my spirit I will be yearning for it even more than I do now."

Many in my congregation were shocked. Many wept. Yet afterward many rethought their priorities in life. They reconsidered their view of their Christian life that now stretched beyond this earth all the way to the eternity and glory of heaven.

More than a few said, "Now I know why my old Christian mother asked me to pray that the Lord would soon take her home. She instinctively knew she was on the edge of the death of her real self. Sad to say, that death occurred long before her physical death."

Still another said, "Now I know that my grandmother's often repeated request that the Lord would take her home was more than just a senile complaint. She wanted to be done with the pain of this earthly life so she could go on and enjoy the blessings of her real heavenly life."

I hope that my prayers and the prayers of my friends are answered so that I will never have to go through death before physical death. However, if this is not God's will, I know that in that hazy suffering I have the assurance of a loving Shepherd who will somehow gently guide me through the black winding terrors of the valley of the shadow of death.

How wonderful it is to be a Christian! How can anyone face life—or death—without Christ?

A NOTE FROM BETTY

Many Christians today are struggling with the problem of euthanasia. Some Christian writers have termed the act of rejecting further medical intervention "passive euthanasia." "Active euthanasia" is normally defined as medical intervention to bring about death as an act of mercy. "Passive euthanasia" is the withholding of nourishment, medications, or mechanical devices that could reasonably be expected to sustain life. It is Bob's and my belief that the patient and his family have the right to determine when further prolonging of the "death process" should be stopped.

Some may say the Bible teaches, "Thou shalt not kill." I agree, but during biblical times the technology to prolong the life or the death process was not available. There came a time when a person could not take nourishment and he said his good-byes and went home to be with the Lord. Today medicine can keep nourishment dripping in, machines breathing for us, and other machines beating our heart for days after even the brain is dead. All of this places a great emotional and financial burden on the family and all of society. Bob and I agree no price is too great to save a life, but this price is too great to prolong the dying.

In Alzheimer's disease, the brain is dying day by day. None of these heroic measures will prolong Bob's "life," only his suffering.

Our agreement now while he is capable of deciding for himself is that death shall be permitted to take its natural course without medical intervention for anything but to maintain what comfort possible. This does not mean we will withhold food and water or regular medications but, rather, when these can no longer be taken willingly they will not be forced by feeding tube or intravenous methods. We have further assured that these wishes will be honored by having an attorney draw up a "Living Will."

TEN
LIFE AFTER LIFE—FROM
MOONLIGHT TO SONLIGHT

I love music. I love the old gospel songs. Since I grew up in the church, I grew up singing. Whether they were able to carry a tune or not, all the people in that country church of my boyhood sang. It was probably by those familiar gospel songs enthusiastically sung by us on Sunday and hummed through the week that we learned our basic theology.

Of all the songs we sang, the happiest and most requested were those about heaven. Songs such as, "When We All Get to Heaven," "O That Will Be Glory," "When the Roll Is Called up Yonder," and "We're Marching to Zion," were sung over and over again. They caused us to focus our attention, not on the cold, dark grave, but instead on that wonderful life that exists beyond our physical life.

Today's children have this same wonderful outlook. By the training of their Sunday school teachers and by the joyfulness of the songs about heaven, they are able to look at life with Jesus as being a continuum—enjoyable now on this earth and continuing in joy in heaven for all eternity.

Because of their great faith and sound theology, little children often have been the great comforters at times of death. During the hundreds of funerals I have conducted, I have often heard little children become the messengers of faith. For instance, I do not know how many times I have heard a little child innocently say, "I can't understand why everyone is crying. After all, grandpa is happy with Jesus in heaven, and pretty soon we will all be happy in heaven with Jesus. Just as soon as we get there, grandpa will be there to hug us." What a silence this produces in a crowd of weeping adults! They look at this innocent four year old with the same awe that they would have for drops of wisdom coming from the great king Solomon. They look at her innocent, trusting face and realize again why Jesus emphasized the pure simple faith of a little child.

In spite of the fact that we use the promise of eternal life as a major benefit to persuade people to make a decision to come to Christ, and in spite of the fact that heaven is the foundation for so many of our happy Christian songs, and in spite of the fact that, to many Christians, heaven is all that makes this earthly life even out and make sense—in spite of all of this, when was the last time you heard a good descriptive sermon about heaven?

The truth of the matter is that ministers are taught almost nothing about heaven during their years of theological training. Thus, you hear more sermons about the Antichrist, death and dying, the tribulation, demonic powers of the underworld, and the phrase "eternal life" than you ever do about heaven itself. Heaven is the foundational expectation of the saints. It deserves a higher recognition than merely to be alluded to during funeral services. Ask your minister to preach a full, scriptural, descriptive sermon about heaven. With today's emphasis on death and the supernatural, Christians have be reminded again and again that death does not end life. There is life after life!

But what kind of life is it? All too often we content ourselves with some sterile statement, such as in the Presbyterian's Westminster Confession of Faith,

> The bodies of men after death return to dust, and seek corruption, but their souls (which neither die nor sleep) having an immortal substance, immediately return to God who gave

them. The souls of the righteous, being then made perfect in holiness, are received into the highest heavens, where they behold the face of God in light and glory, waiting for the full redemption of their bodies; and the souls of the wicked are cast into hell, where they remain in torment and utter darkness, reserved to the judgment of the Great Day. Beside these two places for souls separated from their body, the Scripture acknowledges none.

This is an adequate statement, but certainly not meaningful enough for me as I look toward my heavenly life beginning in a few short years. During this time while I remain here, I can only look forward to my body becoming more painful as it gives up more functions. My spirit will become more agitated, sleepless, and restless. My vision will become distorted as I go into physical as well as mental blackness. My peace will be robbed by those nameless terrors that will come not only at night but also by day.

The total loneliness will drain me as I lose my ability to communicate. Ridiculous agonies will be produced by my confused, tortured mind. The curse of knowing that not only am I totally useless but that I have become a burden to humanity haunts me. The passing from dark moonlight into total blackness in which there is no glimmer of light is a constant fear.

How can I stand to look at this disaster that medical science predicts will most probably overtake me? If I were not a Christian, I do not know how I could stand it. However, since I am a Christian, I can stand it by looking beyond it—looking beyond and considering the glories of heaven where each one of these things will be gone forever to be replaced by perfection, glory, and joy.

Someday my heart will stop beating and my body will be coldly stretched out. Someone unknowingly will say, "Bob Davis is dead."

I am not dead! At the moment my heart stops beating I will at last be fully alive! There is life after life! Scriptures tell us "that to be absent from the body is to be present with the Lord." At last I will be with the Savior I love. At that moment I will be enjoying the fullest dimension of what we dim-sighted earth people called "eternal life."

What will I be experiencing in heaven? Far more than I can ever even dream of now for "eye hath not seen, nor ear heard, neither have entered into the heart of man the things that God has prepared for them that love Him."

Whether all these heavenly blessings will occur in degrees like a flower bud slowly opening to full bloom, or whether they will happen all at once like a burst of color in an aerial fireworks display, I cannot imagine. Although I may not know the time or order of events, I do know from the Bible a few of the blessings I will enjoy.

What do I personally, and every one of Christ's sheep, look forward to? The exhaustion of pain and frustration will be gone and I will instantly experience glorious peace and rest. I will at last have my desperate prayers for rest fully answered as I realize the truth of the verse, "'Blessed are the dead who die in the Lord from now on.' 'Yes,' says the Spirit, 'they will rest from their labor, for their deeds will follow them'" (Rev. 14:13).

This rest will not only relieve my pain-filled body and my terror-filled mind, but it will also relieve my vexed soul. At last I will have rest from sin, wickedness, uncertainty, injustice, and all of the other horrible things that sin produces to ruin man's sojourn on earth. This is not the rest produced by inactivity. Instead it is the rest that comes from being away from the battles that befall the Christian on earth. The burdens of earth are left behind as he enters into that place of completeness in the presence of God and that perfect environment of heaven. At last I will fully leave the moonlight behind forever and be thrilled by the "Sonlight" of heaven. This will come as at last I see the Savior I love face to face, as the songwriter Carrie E. Breck expressed it:

Face to face with Christ my Savior,
Face to face—what will it be—
When with rapture I behold Him,
Jesus Christ who died for me?

Face to face I shall behold Him,
Far beyond the starry sky;
Face to face in all His glory,
I shall see Him by and by!

Painful earth memories will also be removed there. If God did not remove some of our painful earth memories and griefs, heaven could never be heaven for us. Any sadness I have had or tears I have shed will forever be taken away. The Scriptures explain it: "'He will wipe every tear from their eyes. There will be no more death or mourning or crying or pain, for the old order of things has passed away.' He who was seated on the throne said, 'I am making everything new!'" (Rev. 21:4-5). God causes the old things to pass away, and Christ makes all things new . What a glorious promise this is as you couple it with the other benefits of heaven!

We will also have new bodies. What a joy it will be to leave this old, imperfect body behind. The crippled will be made whole, that deformed person made perfect, and that ill person be made new. Benjamin Franklin put it this way in his self-written epitaph. "The body of B. Franklin, printer (like the cover of an old book, its contents torn out and stripped of its lettering and gilding), lies here food for the worm: but the work shall not be lost, for it will (as he believed), appear once more, in a new and more elegant edition, revised and corrected by the author." Crude, but true. In that heavenly day we will have new and more elegant bodies revised and corrected by the Author of Life.

What will our new resurrection body be like? The Bible does not give us any clear answers, but common sense tells us that our bodies will be like the resurrection body of Jesus. After all, we are joint heirs with Christ.

Do you remember what his resurrection body was like? He had a physical body for he let Thomas put his fingers into his nail-pierced hands. He ate. He walked with men on the road to Emmaus, and he looked just like another man to them. But yet it was also a spiritual body. He was instantly transported from place to place. He could pass through solids as if they were nothing, just as when he passed through the barred door into the upper room. And he could cross the miles of space much faster than a slow beam of light for, if you remember, he ascended to heaven and then came back.

What a grand reunion there will be with all the other Christians in heaven! During this earthly time of moonlight, there is a time of loneliness as old friendships gradually grow cold. As my memory fades I can't even remember some of my old friends, let alone talk of some of the precious moments we shared. Through no one's fault, loneliness comes. As we become older we suddenly realize that we have more friends in heaven than we do on earth. We secretly yearn for the old fellowship we enjoyed in better days.

Will we know each other in heaven? Of course we will! In heaven there will be a grand reunion of all the believers we have ever known. There will be our loved ones, our old friends, and all the saints who have gone on before. We will have time to be together. We can love each other deeply without ever grieving over having to say good-bye. We will have all eternity together. We will be forever with the ones we love as well as with every saint who ever lived. Don't forget that we are not speaking about the life span of seventy years. We are speaking about billions of years—eternity if you will!

Certainly, one of the first things we will receive is a new mind. How I long for that! As my mind becomes more confused and forgetful, I long for it to become clear. As I can no longer read and accurately remember I become so frustrated. As my IQ constantly drops I find myself in humiliating circumstances. I yearn to have my old mental pictures and my old memories somehow return. Learning was always such a joy, and I would love to be able to explore new mental paths.

In heaven I will have a new mind in a new and improved version. How many things I want to discover! How many theological questions that I have answered honestly all my life with the short simple statement of, "I don't know," do I want to see unraveled. It will be fun when our faith will be made sight.

Everything in this life stops too short. We are never able to catch up. But there we will have time. We will be able to finish and fulfill our desires there. There will be time to explore the wonders of the universe. How wonderful to know even the simple things of life like how a seed knows which way is up, how a tree knows when to send up sap, or how a spider knows how to spin such a beautifully designed web! Really, doesn't this new dimension of learning sound wonderful?

As I previously mentioned, one of the hardest things that I have ever had to do in my life was to make the transition from one who served to one who had to be served. All of my life I had tried to serve my Lord Jesus Christ. This was my goal, my joy, my satisfaction, and the very purpose, I felt, that God had allowed me to occupy space on planet earth. How deeply I sorrowed when I realized that I could no longer serve Christ! Like so many other things in life, I never really miss it until it is no longer there or no longer possible. I am sure that this is a grief that many other disabled Christians share, a deep grief that those who are functional cannot readily understand.

The Scriptures say, "And his servants will serve him" (Rev. 22:3). Praise the Lord! In my perfected mind and body in heaven, I will again have a way to serve my Lord! I do not know how or why, but again I can do that blessed thing of fully serving Christ my King! What a wonderful thought to fix my mind on as discouragement sometimes makes me wither.

I also expressed my sorrow at not being able to participate in the singing and praise of a worship service. As much as I would like to, I can no longer follow aloud in a unison or responsive reading. Sometimes even the special blessings of a service slip right through my mind. How depressing it is to stand as a mute who cannot think fast enough to join his voice with his fellow Christians in song and praise! I so miss singing!

I personally believe that when we are made complete in heaven that we will have new abilities that are wonderfully magnified. When

I get to heaven I'm going to sing again, sing far better than George Beverly Shea or Caruso ever dreamed of. When you get there, just listen for my new, improved voice!

Thank God, I have a great praise service to look forward to. It will be the greatest praise service ever held, and with my new perfected voice, mind, and body I will fully join in this new song as recorded in Revelation:

> And they sang a new song: "You are worthy to take the scroll and to open its seals, because you were slain, and with your blood you purchased men for God from every tribe and language and people and nation. You have made them to be a kingdom and priests to serve our God, and they will reign on the earth." Then I looked and heard the voice of many angels, numbering thousands upon thousands, and ten thousand times ten thousand. They encircled the throne and the living creatures and the elders. In a loud voice they sang: "Worthy is the Lamb, who was slain, to receive power and wealth and wisdom and strength and honor and glory and praise!" Then I heard every creature in heaven and on earth and under the earth and on the sea, and all that is in them, singing: "To him who sits on the throne and to the Lamb be praise and honor and glory and power, for ever and ever!" (Rev. 5:9-13)

Fellow Christian, have you ever been in a worship service where the joy and praise of the Lord was so great that it seemed to lift you up to heaven? Compared to the joy on that great day in heaven, the joy of your great day on earth will seem like unhappiness. It truly will be joy unspeakable, and full of glory! Even as I think of this, tears come to my eyes and my heart develops a strange homesickness for heaven.

Sheer beauty has always popped into my mind every time I think of heaven. Right now the beautiful pictures and memories in my mind are gone, but I can still go outside and see the beauties of our nature. However, I know that for many of my fellow Alzheimer's sufferers this is a privilege they can no longer enjoy. They are shut up in their rooms, or even bound up in their beds. Some have eyes that can no longer see. Somehow all beauty has faded out of their life during the ravages of this disease.

However, one day beauty will return in a burst of color. We who have trusted Christ will go to be with him and will gasp at this sudden infusion of beauty. How beautiful heaven will be, particularly to those who thought beauty had forever fled from them.

Right now, I walk in partial moonlight. How depressing it would be if all I had to look forward to in life was to journey down into this darkening moonlight only to end up in the cold blackness of the grave. However, I can look beyond the moonlight and see glorious "Sonlight" emanating from the Son of God himself enthroned in that place where all things are changed to become perfect—heaven. This view makes life make sense, gives me patience, and produces a yearning in my heart. The moonlight of my present physical light at times is uncomfortable, but the "Sonlight" in my life to come is glorious. What glory waits for me—in a little while! Isn't it wonderful to be a Christian and to share in the coming glory?

> HEAVEN—just think
> Of stepping on shore,
> And finding it heaven;
> Of taking hold of a hand,
> And finding it God's hand;
> Of breathing new air,
> And finding it heavenly air;
> Of feeling invigorated,
> And finding it immortality;
> Of passing from storm and tempest
> To an unbroken calm;
> Of waking up—
> And finding it HOME!

So my journey goes, from sunlight to moonlight and then to "Sonlight." How wonderful it is to have Jesus as my Shepherd to walk me securely down these paths. Thank God, the journey never ends, but continues until triumph is realized!

"The Spirit and the bride say, 'Come!' And let him who hears say, 'Come!' Whoever is thirsty, let him come; and whoever wishes, let him take the free gift of the water of life" (Rev. 22:17).

EPILOGUE (By Betty)

The disease came like Carl Sandburg's "Fog"—"on little cat feet." The changes were so subtle that they were attributed to "Oh, perhaps his blood sugar is low," or "It's the liver disorder and he just must get more rest." "He's too busy to be held accountable—don't argue with him. When things slow down it will be better." "He is changing—he's getting older and self centered—I am getting old and less attractive—he just doesn't care for me as he did in the hot passion of youth—I am a nuisance rather than a welcomed interruption to his life."

Sometimes I felt sorry that he was under such work pressures—sometimes I just wanted to shake him and say, "What do you mean, you forgot??!!"

Sometimes I feel like God's special pet—held in that special place of all those who are called to share "the fellowship of his suffering." Sometimes I feel like Jesus in the Garden, "Please, if it be your will let this cup pass—let me wake up to learn all this is just a bad dream and all is as before—please come forth in your great healing power God and bring the miracle we've all been praying for and waiting for. Give the literal, physical, renewed mind!"

Sometimes in weakness and despair I want to give voice to that primal scream starting way down in the hidden recesses of the lungs—down where the ever-present knot that lives in my stomach resides—let it whirl through that vortex that's sucking my life and being into the black hole of never-ending pain, emptiness, and loneliness—just give it voice as it rises and explodes through the top of my head—Noooooooooooooo! No, God, no! Not us! Not this! Not his mind! Not his personhood! Anything, God, but this!

Death would be better than this—to hold on to the box when the present is used up—hoping the box can bring again the joy of the reality of the gift—but the box is empty! This is what one has to look forward to with Alzheimer's disease. The body of the one you love—devoid of all expression, of recognition, of joy—here but not here. You are destined to live with only the memory of who he was.

How do you prepare for the holocaust? How can you say good night to your sweetheart and wonder—will this be the night from which reason will never again waken? Will morning find that new person in my bed—the man who will not know who I am or why I am in his bed?

Today we are alive—today we know each other and share simple joys, a walk along the canal, a great blue heron who comes to visit in the backyard, nine peacocks parading past, a little work together, a meal, our memories, many of which I alone hold the key to unlock now. We have set our affairs in order. We have connected ourselves to a good research facility. We have a caring neurologist and internist. We have a supportive local church with many long-time friends. What will we do now? Live, of course.

Live every day to the glory of God. Do every bit of good we can do for as long as we can do it. We have prepared for the worst and now we are going to live expecting the best. If the worst comes we are ready for it. If it doesn't, we will not have wasted today worrying about it.

"This is the day which the Lord hath made; we will rejoice and be glad in it" (Ps. 118:24).